Living with a Sick Child in Hospital

Living with a Sick Child in Hospital

THE EXPERIENCES OF PARENTS AND NURSES

Philip Darbyshire, PhD, MN, RNMH, RSCN, DipN(Lond.), RNT

Senior Lecturer in Health and Nursing Studies, Department of Nursing and Community Health, Glasgow Caledonian University, Glasgow, UK.

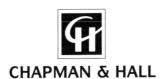

CHAPMAN & HALL

London · Glasgow · Weinheim · New York · Tokyo · Melbourne · Madras

Published by Chapman & Hall,
2–6 Boundary Row, London SE1 8HN, UK

Chapman & Hall, 2–6 Boundary Row, London SE1 8HN, UK

Blackie Academic & Professional, Wester Cleddens Road, Bishopsbriggs, Glasgow G64 2NZ, UK

Chapman & Hall GmbH, Pappelallee 3, 69469 Weinheim, Germany

Chapman & Hall USA, One Penn Plaza, 41st Floor, New York NY 10119, USA

Chapman & Hall Japan, ITP-Japan, Kyowa Building, 3F, 2-1-1 Hirakawacho, Chiyoda-ku, Tokyo 102, Japan

Chapman & Hall Australia, Thomas Nelson Australia, 102 Dodds Street, South Melbourne, Victoria 3205, Australia

Chapman & Hall India, R. Seshadri, 32 Second Main Road, CIT East, Madras 600 035, India

Distributed in the USA and Canada by Singular Publishing Group Inc., 4284 41st Street, San Diego, California 92105, USA

First edition 1994

© 1994 Chapman & Hall

Typeset in 10/12 Times by Florencetype Ltd, Kewstoke, Avon
Printed in Great Britain

ISBN   0 412 61050 7   1 56593 374 5 (USA)

A catalogue record for this book is available from the British Library

Library of Congress Cataloging-in-Publication data available

♾ Printed on permanent acid-free text paper, manufactured in accordance with ANSI/NISO Z39.48-1992 and ANSI/NISO Z39.48-1984 (Permanence of Paper).

To my wife Hilary and my daughter Emma,
whose ways of 'being-in-the-world'
constantly remind me that these
are no abstract concepts.

Contents

Foreword: parenting in public by Patricia Benner   xi
Preface   xiii
Acknowledgements   xv
Notation used in interview transcription   xvi
Introduction   xvii

**1   Parents, nurses and paediatric nursing:
a review of the literature**   1

1.1   Introduction   1
    1.1.1 The historical context   2
    1.1.2 Parental involvement and participation   6
    1.1.3 Nurses and live-in parents   9
    1.1.4 Parents' accounts   14

1.2   Summary and conclusions   15

2   Becoming a live-in parent: 'parenting in public'   17

2.1   Introduction   17
    2.1.1 Parents' reasons for wishing to live-in   18
       (a) Circumstantial reasons   18
       (b) Instrumental reasons   18
       (c) Protective and advocacy reasons   19
       (d) Emotional and supportive reasons   19
    2.1.2 Deciding to live-in   20
    2.1.3 Admission: becoming 'a different parent'   23
    2.1.4 Parental uncertainty: the 'emotional roller-coaster'   25
    2.1.5 Concluding comments   31

2.2   Adapting to becoming a live-in parent   33
    2.2.1 Sharing responsibility and care   33
    2.2.2 Discipline: 'trying to get back to normal'   35
    2.2.3 'Learning the ropes'   37
    2.2.4 Concluding comments   40

2.3 Nurses' perceptions of live-in parents   40
    2.3.1 Nurses' expectations: co-operation, competence
        and character   41
    2.3.2 Creating parents and family   46
        (a) Marginalized family: being 'out of it'   49
        (b) Who are 'family' in family-centred care?   50
    2.3.3 Concluding comments   52

2.4 Summary   53

3 The moral imperative: being a 'good parent'   55

3.1 Introduction   55
    3.1.1 Establishing a moral purpose   56
    3.1.2 Being guilty   57

3.2 Establishing and re-establishing moral identities   60
    3.2.1 Defensive parenting: being 'in the presence of experts' 60
    3.2.2 Showing an interest   62
    3.2.3 Avoiding social activities   63
    3.2.4 Pulling your weight   64
    3.2.5 Not being a nuisance   66
    3.2.6 Being competent   67

3.3 Nurses and parents' moral identities   69
    3.3.1 Creating parents' moral identities   69
    3.3.2 Judging the judgers?   72
    3.3.3 Getting to know the person of the parent   75

3.4 Concluding comments   80

4 Parental involvement and participation   83

4.1 Introduction   83

4.2 Parents' experiences of participation   84
    4.2.1 Determining participation: parents' understandings 84
    4.2.2 Parents and play: 'worse than working'   89
    4.2.3 Basic mothering: doing 'the natural mother things' 93
    4.2.4 Technical tasks: 'the medical things'   94
    4.2.5 Keeping vigil   97
    4.2.6 Breaks and meals: 'no rest for the wicked'   99
    4.2.7 Summary   103

4.3 Nurses and the creation of parent participation   104
    4.3.1 Parent participation: nurses' understandings and practices 104
    4.3.2 Parent participation and the demarcation of care 109
    4.3.3 Nurses and the unspoken arrangement   110

(a) The inform-and-leave strategy 111
(b) The as-if-at-home analogy 113
4.3.4 Nurses and the expert parent 115

4.4 Concluding comments 117

5 Parents' and nurses' relationships 120

5.1 Introduction 120

5.2 Parents' perceptions of nurses and nursing 120
5.2.1 The nurses' work 120
5.2.2 Nurses as perpetually busy 122
5.2.3 The value of nurses' caring practices 125
5.2.4 The absence and breakdown of caring practices 129

5.3 The developing relationship between parents and nurses 133
5.3.1 Initial encounters 133
5.3.2 From professional and parent to 'a special relationship' 135

5.4 Nurses' relationships with live-in parents 137
5.4.1 Creating the relationship: connecting with parents 137
5.4.2 Initial encounters and intuitive assessments 139
5.4.3 Having sustained contact with parents 141
5.4.4 Parents who were 'in too long' 144

5.5 Parents' other lives: families and homes 146
5.5.1 The support of family and friends 146
5.5.2 Maintaining home and family connections 147
5.5.3 Coping with the demands of families and friends 150

5.6 Relationships between parents: alone together 152
5.6.1 Parents' shared concerns and identities: 'all in the same boat'? 153
5.6.2 Difficulties experienced in relationships between parents 159

5.7 Concluding comments 162

6 Concluding discussion 165

6.1 Introduction 165

6.2 The research philosophy and approach reviewed 165

6.3 Major themes of the study 166
6.3.1 The nature of being a live-in parent in hospital 166
(a) The ontological sense of being a live-in parent 166
(b) The situated meaning of being a live-in parent 168
(c) Being in the situation: involvement and control 171
6.3.2 Parents and nurses: caring and relationships 176

(a) Caring as a human trait? 176
(b) Caring as a moral imperative or ideal? 177
(c) Caring as the nurse–parent relationship? 178
6.3.3 Caring as a fusion of concerns 180

6.4 Implications 182

7 The research approach and methods 186

7.1 The purpose and focus of the study 186
7.1.1 The purpose of the study 186
7.1.2 Research approach and methods 187
7.1.3 The focus of the study 187
7.1.4 The selection of a qualitative design 188

7.2 Theoretical underpinnings of the study 189
7.2.1 The combining of complementary approaches 189
7.2.2 Phenomenology 190
7.2.3 Grounded theory 191
7.2.4 The assumptions of grounded theory and phenomenology 191

7.3 The research method 193
7.3.1 The setting 193
7.3.2 Selecting the research participants 195
7.3.3 The parents 195
7.3.4 The children 196
7.3.5 The nurses 196

7.4 Obtaining the accounts 196
7.4.1 Bracketing, guiding and generative questions 197
7.4.2 Engaging the participants' involvement 197
7.4.3 The interviews 199
7.4.4 Ethical considerations 200
7.4.5 Interpretive analysis 204
7.4.6 Rigour and trustworthiness 205

7.5 Concluding comments 206

References 208
Index 221

Foreword: parenting in public

This book is remarkable for its honesty and unflinching dialogue about the everyday relational ethics of parents and nurses engaged in the fragile enterprise of caring for acutely ill children in public hospitals. Philip Darbyshire's research enters the everyday worlds of parents and sick children as experienced and understood in the midst of suffering and vulnerability. What he finds there are core existential meanings and moral visions of what it means to be a parent. Dr Darbyshire calls our attention to the distinctions between public and private lives in the most intimate and vulnerable situation of having one's taken-for-granted caring relationships scrutinized and 'managed'.

He pulls back the veils of our elaborate systems of explanation, therapeutic notions, control and power and allows the reader to see with him how these are manifested in the first-hand experience of parents and nurses. We see pervasive meanings and visions of parenting exposed in the institutional structures and practices of caring for acutely ill children and infants. The cultural confusion between care and control becomes painfully clear as advice and management are more easily actualized than care and compassion.

The moral emotions of shame, blame, guilt and responsibility are heard and retold in particular voices and particular stories. Dr Darbyshire resists the temptation to 'cope' with the stories through additional explanations. He stands alongside the parents and nurses and hears the competing goods, the anguish and the moral turpitude that occur in the face of sorrow and suffering. The aim of the work is increased understanding of, and compassion for, parents, children and nurses. He enters the realm of the ethics of relationships without moralizing.

In the 'business' of hospitals, much has been made about understanding the hospital encounter from the 'customer's' perspective. What this consumerism ignores is the way in which patients or the parents of sick children are not willing customers choosing hospital services, but, rather, horrified, unwilling entrants whose world is threatened. This work carefully reveals the everyday world of parents of sick or injured children in the hospital doing what they can and must do as their worlds are irrevocably changed. We experience the institutions that challenge, chide, confront and sometimes care for vulnerable parents. We see our unwitting systems of exclusion and blame. The nurse's vantage point is also presented. Existential, relational and structural meanings of living in the public hospital are examined. We find that the units are set up for mothers rather than fathers and that the nurses are more at home than the parents and patients.

This is a profound work calling for a revolution of the heart, mind and care-giving practices. It offers a practical approach to the everyday ethics of relation-ships. Those who are concerned about biomedical ethics would do well to look here for a fresh start. This work is a brilliant example of the ethics of care and responsiveness.

We have created elaborate systems of judgments that allow us to flee from the vulnerability and unthinkable suffering, neglect, cruelty and death of our children. We cover over, with technique and institutional responses, the awesome social responsibility of **being** parents as opposed to 'doing parenting'. Philip Darbyshire's work calls us to reconnect with these more primordial issues and take better care of one another by listening, standing alongside – in short – by caring. I commend this book to all care-givers, professional and lay. If we listen to the voices here, we will gain new visions of how to design our institutions of public care-giving.

Patricia Benner
March 1994

Preface

PARENTING IN PUBLIC: PARENTS, HOSPITALS AND NURSES

Since the publication of the Platt Report of 1959 into the welfare of children in hospital, there has been increasing concern among parents, professionals and policy makers concerning how we might 'humanize' the experience of hospitalization for children and their families.

A variety of strategies have been advocated and adopted throughout the UK, and in other countries, in order to achieve this goal. A central strategy here has been to encourage parents to 'live-in' with their child during their stay in hospital, and to participate more fully in their child's care.

However, the research literature suggests that this thrust towards parental living-in and increased participation has occurred more at the level of official and professional ideology than in everyday practice. There has been a distinct lack of work that asks parents about the nature of this experience of living-in with their hospitalized child. Similarly, the other vital players in this strategy, the children's nurses, have been overlooked with the result that our understandings of if and how nurses make 'parental involvement and participation' work in practice are scant.

This book is based on my recent doctoral research study which examined and described in detail the experiences both of parents and of nurses in relation to many crucial aspects of paediatric hospitalization.

In this book I explore fundamental issues regarding the nature of being the parent of a hospitalized child and a children's nurse. It shows how currently cherished policy objectives of parent participation, living-in and family-centred care are significantly more problematic than has previously been assumed.

The current health-care climate stresses increasing 'consumer' involvement and increasing participation and partnership in health care. While such a strong emphasis is currently being placed on quality in health-care provision, it seems vital that in order to provide a responsive, quality service for the 1990s and beyond, we must have a much greater understanding of the actual lived experiences of both the parents of the hospitalized child and their nurses. I believe that this book promotes such a deeper understanding.

This book has practical implications for both children's nurses and those involved in formulating policy for children's health care. Numerous 'everyday' and 'taken for granted' aspects of hospital care are shown to be much more complex than has been traditionally assumed. These issues are highlighted particularly memorably and graphically in the presented accounts and narratives of both parents and nurses.

These narratives and accounts of the lived experience of parents and nurses are used to suggest ways in which nurses can use their own stories in order to reflect more meaningfully on their practice. For those involved in preparing children and parents for a period of hospitalization, the book offers much rich description of how parents actually experience the process of being with their hospitalized child.

Hospital and nurse managers will discover much about what parents look for from the health-care system in order to help them through this most traumatic of experiences.

As a nurse educator, I am aware that educationalists are often challenged by how best to prepare nurses to work empathetically with parents and families. This book offers numerous critique points within which to engage students in discussion of salient issues such as 'parent participation', 'family-centred care', 'standards', 'nurse–parent relationships' and the primacy of 'caring' in nursing. The parents' vivid descriptions of nurses and nursing practices that they found to be both helpful and unhelpful will be welcomed by nurse teachers interested in promoting effective and valuable nurse caring.

The material published here also appeared in a similar form as Darbyshire, P. (1990) Parenting in public, in *Advances in Child Health Nursing*, (eds E.A. Glasper and A. Tucker), Scutari Press, London, p. 247–256. I am grateful to Scutari Press for their permission to draw on this material for this book.

Acknowledgements

This book is based upon my PhD thesis. The study was made possible by the award of a Scottish Home and Health Department Nursing Research Training Fellowship which I held from 1986–1989, based at the Nursing Research Unit, Department of Nursing Studies, University of Edinburgh. Without such sustained financial and scholarly support, my interest in this subject may have remained a series of unexamined hunches.

My supervisors, Dr Alison Tierney and Helen Sinclair were critical, encouraging and supportive in exactly the right measure. Their understandings of the peaks and troughs of research led me back to thinking when I thought that I had found 'the answer' in only my second draft and helped me see good in the study when I could see precious little.

Research is often characterized as a solitary venture. This notion, however, does scant justice to the reality of sustaining and completing a study. Friends and colleagues play a larger part in a study than they perhaps realize. Steve Tilley provided the encouragement of tough questions, staff at Glasgow Caledonian University encouraged and enabled me to 'finish that thesis', Martha MacLeod remains a good friend and invaluable spur to thinking from as far away as Canada and Rosemary Morris at Chapman & Hall has believed in this study almost since its beginnings. My debt to Patricia Benner and her scholarship is apparent throughout this book.

My wife Hilary and daughter Emma have also lived with this study. To say that 'I couldn't have done it without them' would only trivialize the extent of their support.

My greatest thanks are of course to the study participants. The senior hospital staff, both nursing and medical, made 'research access' a pleasure rather than an ordeal and could not have been more welcoming or supportive. Ward staff were equally accepting of my presence and keen to share their stories and experiences with me. The parents were unstinting in sharing their experiences with me and I am all the more appreciative for knowing that they did this during some of the most traumatic and taxing times of their lives.

Notation used in interview transcription

The interviews were transcribed verbatim. Facilitative sounds, e.g. 'Uhuh', to encourage a participant to carry on are not generally included, nor were 'errs' and 'ums' where these were simply participants pausing or hesitating while speaking. Much as I love the richness of Scots dialect, I have at least partially 'anglicized' some of the words and expressions used by the participants in the interests of wider understanding.

The following notation is used in direct participant quotations:

PD: Philip Darbyshire, the interviewer. The participants are referred to as Nurse A, Mother, etc.

1, Mother 1 or Nurse 1: Refers to a particular participant in a focus group discussion.

...: A pause in the interview. Two or more sets of these dots indicate a proportionally longer pause.

(...): I have edited a section of the interview.

[words]: I have added some explanatory or supplementary note or comment.

(word): Indicates a participant's response, e.g. (laughs).

bold text: Participant's emphasis., unless otherwise stated.

Note: References given after the transcriptions, e.g. (26, Mother 4, p. 2), refer to the author's original notes.

Introduction

'If you take away a sick child from the parents or nurse you break its heart immediately'. So warned Dr George Armstrong, a noted 18th-century physician (cited by Miles, 1986a, p. 83) Now in the late 20th century the desirability of encouraging parents to live-in with their hospitalized child is widely accepted. The latest UK government report, *Welfare of Children and Young People in Hospital* (Department of Health, 1991, p. 16), states that 'a cardinal principle of hospital services for children is complete ease of access to the child by his parents, and to other members of the family (as well as a mother or father "a parent" could be a grandparent, uncle, aunt, sibling, nanny or close friend of the family). This is not a luxury'. The report also stresses that 'good child health care is shared with partners/carers and they are closely involved in the care of their children at all times, unless exceptionally this is not in the best interests of their child' (Department of Health, 1991, p. 2).

This was not always so and the history of paediatric care is one where improvements in child health existed side-by-side with a disregard for this 'human' side of child and family care which seems almost barbaric today. In this book I explore the meaning of these 'cardinal principles' in practice.

Resident parents and paediatric nurses have been relatively ignored, compared for example with the body of research on hospitalization and children. As a result, we have scant understanding of how parents experience living-in with their hospitalized child or how paediatric nurses practise within the expressed philosophy of family-centred care.

This lack of understanding is untenable in today's health-care climate where the public are less and less likely to tolerate what they perceive to be unacceptable standards of care. The watchwords of our times are 'accountability', 'effectiveness' 'efficiency', 'quality' and partnership with our 'consumers'. If we are to provide paediatric care which respects the 'cardinal principles' of parental access and participation that truly meet the needs of parents and children, then we must plan and deliver services which are based upon a much clearer understanding of 'what this is like' for parents. This involves considerably more than devising slick 'customer pleasing' strategies and adding a few reassuring phrases to the glossy corporate brochure or 'mission statement'.

We need to go to those participants most closely involved in 'family-centred care', that is live-in parents and paediatric nurses, to discover the meanings, understandings and implications of such rhetoric in practice. We then need to consider how best to enable practitioners and parents to create the kind of partnerships which cannot be enforced by memo or fiat.

The structure of the book is as follows. In Chapter 1 I trace the historical development of parental involvement in paediatrics. The literature reviewed shows that parental participation and living-in have been seen as essentially unproblematic, both philosophically and professionally. The 'cardinal principles' of parental access and involvement have been advocated and operationalized with little or no attempt made to try to understand what living-in is like for either parents or nurses.

In Chapters 2 to 5 I present and explore the major themes that arose from the participants' interview accounts and fieldwork conversations. Chapter 2 examines how parents became live-in parents in what is a very public arena, looking particularly at their experiences during the early period of hospitalization. Nurses' understandings of resident parents are also presented and I examine how the social phenomenon of live-in parents is co-created.

In Chapter 3, I show that being a live-in parent is as much a moral as a practical endeavour in that parents feel a need to establish their moral identities as 'good parents' within the context of the ward. I also show the nurses' influences in shaping parents' moral identity.

Chapter 4 examines the major theme of parental participation and involvement. Participants' accounts illuminate this complex aspect of paediatric hospitalization, showing that this is more problematic and multidimensional than has previously been acknowledged.

In Chapter 5 the nature of the relationship between live-in parents and nurses is explored. Participants' accounts reveal that this relationship is dynamic, fluid and multifaceted. The parents' accounts also stress the vital importance of nurses' caring practices in helping mutually satisfying relationships to develop.

Chapter 6 reviews the major themes and develops a further interpretative analysis of the ontological meaning of being a live-in parent and of the concept of caring which was fundamental to the nurse–parent relationship. I also outline what I believe to be the major implications of this study for nursing research, education and practice.

Finally, Chapter 7 gives a detailed account of the research approach and methods used in this study. I have purposely placed this chapter at the end of the book because much as it troubles some researchers, research methods chapters are not every reader's idea of an appetizing and stimulating start to a book. This aside, there is an assured need to include such research details in a book reporting the findings of a study. To truly understand the context of the study and to evaluate its ethics, rigour and trustworthiness, the reader must be able to see where the data and interpretations have 'come from' and how they have been handled. I hope that this chapter might also be useful in helping other researchers who might be planning a similar type of qualitative study.

Parents, nurses and paediatric nursing: a review of the literature | 1

1.1 INTRODUCTION

Hospitalization has long been recognized as being a potentially stressful time for both children and their parents. Stimulated by the influential work of James and Joyce Robertson in the late 1950s and early 1960s (Robertson, 1970; Robertson and Robertson, 1989), research on the hospitalized child has tended to focus on issues related to separation and the possibility of adverse effects on the child either in the short or long term (Fletcher, 1981). Since the publication of the Platt Report (Ministry of Health, 1959), there have been attempts to humanize paediatric hospitals by offering open visiting (Fagin and Nusbaum, 1978), living-in facilities for parents (Hardgrove, 1980) and by encouraging parents to take a more active part in their child's care while in hospital (Sainsbury *et al.*, 1986; Cleary *et al.*, 1986).

However, there is evidence to suggest that while such changes may be desirable, their implementation has been more difficult than was first imagined (Consumers Association, 1980; Hall, 1978; 1987). Hospitals are complex environments and the phrase 'encourage parents to live-in with their child' tends to underestimate the implications of this increased parental presence for both parents and paediatric nurses (Elfert and Anderson, 1987; Hall, 1987).

Throughout the literature on paediatric hospitalization there is a lack of detailed description as to how parents and nurses perceive these changes. The questions 'How do parents experience living-in with their child in a paediatric ward?' and 'What is the nature of nurses' relationships with live-in parents?' have remained unanswered and largely unasked.

Clearly, the body of literature on children in hospital is too vast to be comprehensively reviewed. It is more valuable here to selectively focus upon those aspects of paediatric hospitalization that consider parents' and nurses' experiences, particularly where this relates to parents who live-in with their child. I begin by tracing an outline of the changes in philosophies of paediatric care that have taken place this century. This provides a context within which to discuss the more germane aspects of parental living-in, parental involvement and participation in the child's care and the nature of the nurse–parent relationship.

1.1.1 The historical context

Hospitals for sick children are comparatively new institutions, emerging mainly in the mid-19th century (Miles, 1986a). Prior to this there existed dispensaries that gave advice and medicine to parents who called. The first of these was opened by Dr George Armstrong in 1769. Dr Armstrong believed that children should not be separated from their parents and admitted to hospital, claiming prophetically that 'the mothers and the nurses would be constantly at variance with each other' (Miles, 1986a, p. 83). The major task of these new hospitals was to deal with the range of illnesses, mostly infectious and deficiency diseases, that were so much the products of the social conditions of the time. Indeed initially, Great Ormond Street Hospital in London barred children who had accidents or external injuries (Miles, 1986a, p. 85). This early struggle against infectious diseases and often fatal illnesses helped to create a hospital system based upon asepsis and rigid following of routine. The legacy of this system was to affect the relationships between children, their parents and hospital staff for over a century and its last vestiges may even be apparent today.

The ethos of child care within the paediatric hospitals was not shaped solely by physical factors. The child-rearing ideologies of the early 20th century provided further justification for mechanistic and regimented care. Hardyment (1983) showed that the prevailing orthodoxy of the time regarding relationships with children was one of firm, cold detachment. Child care experts of the 1920s and 1930s such as Truby King advocated the strictest adherence to 'by-the-clock' routine, while the celebrated behaviourist J. B. Watson advised mothers:

> Never hug or kiss them. Never let them sit on your lap. If you must, kiss them once on the forehead when they say goodnight. Shake hands with them in the morning. Give them a pat on the head if they have made an extremely good job of a difficult task. Try it out. In a week's time you will find how easy it is to be perfectly objective with your child and at the same time kindly. You will be ashamed of the mawkish, sentimental way you have been handling it. (Cited in Hardyment, 1983, p. 175)

With the decline in infectious diseases, and the introduction of antibiotics and technological innovations, these patterns of child care might have been expected to disappear. However, it was changes in thinking concerning the child's psychological and emotional development that were to be the most effective catalysts for change.

Several paediatricians began to promote schemes that kept mothers and children together. Sir James Spence established a small mother and baby unit in 1927 at the Babies Hospital in Newcastle-upon-Tyne (Spence, 1946). In New Zealand, in the 1940s, Pickerill and Pickerill (1946; 1954) admitted mothers to help care for their child on a plastic surgery unit and reported that, contrary to the received view of the time, there was no increase in cross-infection rates due to the mothers' presence. At Amersham Hospital in the UK, paediatrician Dermot MacCarthy and Ward Sister Ivy Morris were pioneering liberal paediatric care practices which 'anticipated the recommendations of the Platt Report'. (Robertson and Robertson, 1989, p. 59)

Many regard the watershed events regarding care of the hospitalized child as being the work of John Bowlby (1953) and James Robertson (1962; 1970). Bowlby's highly influential work on 'maternal deprivation' was seen as being particularly applicable to the situation of the hospitalized child. The Robertsons' films of children undergoing hospitalization and separation had a dramatic effect on professional and public opinion. Viewers were confronted with the sight of the emotional disintegration of children in places where they were ostensibly there to be helped. The impact of films such as *John: Nine Days in a Residential Nursery* and *A Two-Year-Old Goes to Hospital* was enhanced by the Robertsons' stark, almost telegrammatic commentary which did attract criticism from professionals for being 'subjective' (Hawthorne, 1974; p. 21). However, such critics declined to suggest how the documentary pain and distress of a child could be commented upon objectively.

The importance and impact of this work are hard to over-estimate. Today's audiences watching films like *A Two-Year-Old Goes to Hospital* usually find it hard to believe that paediatric 'care' was ever actually like this. What seems equally unbelievable today is the extent and ferocity of the paediatric medical establishment's critical reactions to this film. Hawthorne (1974, p. 19) would have us believe that the critics merely 'doubted the validity' of the film and says that it met with 'some scepticism'. However a more realistic Robertson details the reception of the film (Robertson and Robertson, 1989, p. 43–51, describing how he was vilified by audiences of paediatricians and nurses across the country as he showed the film in their hospitals.

The criticisms were as absurd as they were defensive: the child filmed was 'atypical', she was never filmed when she was 'happy', the editing was selective, the nurses had been deliberately prevented from playing with and comforting her by Robertson himself, but most commonly, that no such unhappy, distressed child had ever been seen in **their** hospital. NIMBY-ism with a vengeance. Even the supposedly 'liberal' Sir James Spence was 'caustically negative as before and his lieutenants followed his lead' (Robertson and Robertson, 1989, p. 45).

During this period, some paediatric nurses began to advocate more humane and family-focused practices such as allowing parents to visit their hospitalized child. Duncombe, in an article in *Nursing Times* (1951, p. 587) wrote of the 'arguments against daily visiting that I hear again and again both in personal conversation and at professional meetings'. In the present era, it is difficult to comprehend that the position that she was defending against such entrenched criticism was that of allowing parents to visit their child for 'one planned half-hour a day'.

Although telling accounts of the visitation struggles of parents of the time have been compiled (Robertson, 1962), perhaps the most vivid account of how 'the system' conspired against parents is a literary one, in Margaret Drabble's book, *The Millstone*. Set in this period of late 1950s–early 1960s, it features a section where the central character, Rosamund Stacey's, baby daughter Octavia has to be admitted to hospital:

> When I went round in the morning to visit her, I found myself met by a certain unhelpful stalling. The lady in charge, a lady in white whose title was not clear to me, assured me that all was well, that all was progressing most satisfactorily, that the child was as comfortable as could be expected. 'I'd like to go and see her,' I said then, summoning up a little courage.
>
> 'I'm afraid that won't be possible,' said the lady in white with a calm certainty, looking down at her file of notes.
>
> 'Why not?' I said. 'I would like to see her, I know she'd like to see me.'
>
> The lady in white embarked upon a long explanation about upsetting children, upsetting mothers, upsetting other children, upsetting other mothers, justice to all, disturbing the nurses' routine, and such topics. (. . .) 'What about visiting hours?' I said, and back came the civil, predictable answer, 'I'm afraid that for such small infants we don't allow any visiting at all. We really do find that it causes more inconvenience to staff and patients than we can possibly cope with. Really, Mrs Stacey, you must understand that it is of no practical use to visit such a young child, she will settle much more happily if she doesn't see you. You'd be amazed to see how soon they settle down. Mothers never believe us, but we know from experience how right we are to make this regulation.' (Drabble, 1965, p. 148–149)

Eventually, Rosamund is driven to shouting and screaming as the 'lady in white' is forcibly leading her out of the ward. Only through this 'making a huge fuss' is she at last allowed to see her child.

Real life for parents could however be much more tragic than fiction. While James Robertson's films were visual stimuli for change, one parent's voice provided an equally unanswerable case for humane access. In 1965, two noted paediatricians, Dermot MacCarthy and Ronald MacKeith, published 'A Parent's Voice' in the *Lancet* (1965) and again, 20 years later, in *Archives of Disease in Childhood* (1985). In this short, heartbreaking letter, a mother told of how her three-year-old daughter, Dawn, who had 'never been anywhere without me' had been admitted to hospital for tonsillectomy and adenoidectomy. Dawn began crying almost as soon as her mother had to leave. Her mother was not allowed to visit on the day of surgery but could telephone. When she phoned at midday, Dawn was fine but 'no' she still could not visit, but she could phone again at 6 pm. When she phoned again at 6 pm she was told that Dawn was haemorrhaging but 'not to worry'. Again, she was not allowed to visit. Dawn's mother continues:

Thursday, 18th, 10.30 am. I telephoned the hospital, spoke to the ward sister and was told that Dawn was a little improved and that I could visit at 4 o'clock. I arrived at the hospital at 3.50 pm and was asked to wait because the doctor was with Dawn. A few minutes later I was told that Dawn had collapsed but not to worry because the doctor was doing all possible. I asked if I could go to her but was told to wait. As I waited I prayed to God to help my little girl; a few minutes later the ward sister came and said that my dear Dawn had passed away at 4.15 pm, so you see although I was there I couldn't go in to see her even though she was dying. They took me to see Dawn then but it was too late for my love to do its work because she had gone to rest.

A *Nursing Times* editorial of the time was highly critical of the restrictions that kept parents and their children apart. It noted that 'in the Annual Report for the Ministry (of Health) for 1952, tables showed that 141 hospitals under regional hospital boards and three teaching hospitals prohibited the visiting of children except in emergency' (*Nursing Times* Editorial, 1953, p. 1153).

Paediatric nurses in the USA at this time were also writing in their nursing journals, describing how they were influenced by psychological theories of separation and how they were trying to encourage contact between the hospitalized child and their parents (Frank, 1952; Morgan and Lloyd, 1955; Hartrich, 1956; Hohle, 1957).

The major impetus towards reuniting parents with their hospitalized child came with the publication of the Platt Report (*The Welfare of Children in Hospital*, Ministry of Health, 1959) and in subsequent DHSS memoranda that stressed the importance of open visiting. The central thrust of the Platt Report was that greater heed had to be taken of the hospitalized child's emotional and psychological welfare. This was to be achieved through the report's major recommendations. These were:

- that alternatives to in-patient treatment should be available;
- that children should be admitted to children's hospitals or wards;
- that children's nurses should be specifically trained;
- that parents should be able to visit at any 'reasonable' time of day or night; and
- that organized play and recreational activities should be provided in each ward.

The fate of the Platt Report is perhaps best understood in the light of Florence Nightingale's observation that 'reports are not necessarily self-executive'. Progress in implementing the recommendations of the Platt Report was slow and varied greatly across the country (Rodgers, 1980; Consumers Association, 1980; Swanwick, 1983). Government inaction was limited to the issuing of a succession of circulars that could only advise. Sixteen years after Platt, the Court Report (*Fit For the Future*, Department of Health and Social Security, 1976, p. 190) was still able to note that 'a great deal of evidence we received underlined the fact that it is in the sphere of social understanding of their needs that children are least well cared for (. . .) our visits made it clear that the personal needs of children in acute hospitals were not being met.'

In 1961 a group of parents formed NAWCH (National Association for the Welfare of Children in Hospital), now called Action for Sick Children. For the last 30 years NAWCH has monitored and reported on how the spirit and the recommendations of the Platt Report have been put into practice throughout the country. In relation to parental access to their child, NAWCH has reported that, in England, children were still being admitted to adult wards where visiting restrictions were greater than in paediatric wards and to ENT wards which had many more visiting and parental restrictions than other paediatric wards (Thornes, 1983a).

Thornes (1983b) also found wide variations in access; for example only 21% of wards in the Northern Region allowed unrestricted access compared with 82% in North East Thames Region. In a similar Scottish study, Wolfe (1985) found that 61% claimed to have unrestricted access for parents, although 9% restricted parental visits on operating day. Sixteen of the wards could not or would not accommodate parents overnight.

Hall (1978) argued that the slow and piecemeal implementation of the Platt Report's recommendations was due to the fact that Platt had considered only psychological theory, that is mother–child separation. Hall believed that they had ignored the wider sociological implications of hospitals as institutions and the difficulty inherent in effecting change within such places. Hall (1978) also argued that having parents in the ward as visitors or residents created resistance from staff who did not accept either that parents should be there or the evidence showing that parental presence was a good thing.

There seemed little doubt that the Platt Report's analyses of the problem and suggested solutions were rather narrow in vision and naive in expectation. Parents were encouraged to stay with their child during their hospitalization, either as 'long-term' and regular visitors or as residents. What had not been seriously considered was how parents and nurses would experience this living-in, what would be expected of them and what effect would such living-in have upon their respective child-care and nursing practices.

1.1.2 Parental involvement and participation

The literature on parent participation from both the UK and North America suggests that this is one of paediatric nursing's most amorphous and ill-described concepts. Parents and nurses seem to have different attitudes toward the concept, different ideas as to what the term actually means and different notions as to what parental participation involves in the daily life of a children's ward. In an influential study Meadow (1969) described the lives of live-in parents under the graphic title of 'The Captive Mother'. He suggested that such parents were akin to prisoners in that they were confined, not by bars but by expectations and a sense of anomie. The parents described their situation as being primarily one of boredom where their role was merely to sit by the bedside while having little or no involvement in their child's care.

Several other studies at this time showed that mothers were keen to have a more active participatory role in the care of their child. Beck (1973) surveyed 38 parents to ascertain their attitudes towards a 'patient care unit' or what would now be called a Care By Parent Unit (Green and Green, 1977; Monaghan and Schkade, 1985; Sainsbury *et al.*, 1986) where parents have responsibility for providing their child's daily care with available guidance and support from nurses. While the parents felt comfortable about carrying out aspects of care such as giving emotional support, accompanying the child for tests and feeding and changing, they were unsure as to their own ability to carry out more technical or procedural care such as the recording of vital signs or helping to administer medications. The reasons that they gave for this suggested a compromised self-confidence and sense of competence. They were unwilling to upset the hospital routine and 'get in the way' and were also wary of making a mistake.

Jackson *et al.* (1978) determined parents' desire for participation on admission to hospital with a view to sharing this information with the ward nursing staff. Of the 31 parents questioned, 'the overwhelming majority wanted to participate in their child's care, and for the most part they wanted to do so without the aid of a nurse'. Again, most parents wished to participate in emotional and supportive and nurturing tasks with fewer parents wishing to be involved in technical and procedural activities. The questionnaire used initially was completed by parents three days after their admission and it was found that changes that occurred were 'in the direction of more independence over time', especially in relation to a greater willingness to perform more 'medically orientated activities'.

An earlier study by Merrow and Johnson (1968) suggested discrepancies between mothers and paediatric nurses regarding 'what a mother would like her own role to be with her hospitalized child'. Fifty nurses and 50 parents were given a questionnaire to complete concerning the carrying out of various child-care tasks in the ward. The researchers concluded that 'in most instances the mothers preferred to be responsible for more aspects of their child's care than the paediatric nurses realized'. This finding has been supported by other studies, for example Webb *et al.* (1985) and, more recently, Brown and Ritchie (1990).

Several studies found that parents were generally keen to participate and be involved in their child's care. In a study of 76 parents of non-seriously-ill children, MacDonald (1969) found that over 90% of the parents were willing to carry out nurturing, encouraging and washing and feeding tasks. While mothers were willing to participate in various areas of care, Hawthorne (1974, p. 133), for example, found that nurses were much more inclined to encourage parents to become involved in 'basic nursing tasks' (*sic*) such as washing, feeding and changing the child. Hawthorne (1974, p. 133) also reported an 'overwhelming reluctance' on the part of nurses to allow parents to participate in any nursing care which 'might be described in any way as technical nursing'. Hill (1978) interviewed 18 mothers whose children 'were not seriously ill, unconscious or handicapped', (the researcher did not detail diagnoses), regarding their participation in four categories of care: stimulation and entertainment, comfort measures, activities of daily living and therapeutic measures. It was found that an overall 78% of the mothers wanted to participate in their child's care. Hill noted that over 90% of the mothers wanted to participate mainly in comfort and stimulation and entertainment work while only 61% were keen to become involved in more technical and medical routines. As part of the 'Swansea studies' – see also Stacey, Hall, Pill, Jacobs – a programme of studies into children in hospital carried out in the late 1960s and 1970s, Jacobs (1979, p. 102) observed that 'little attempt was made by hospital staff to involve parents in ward life while they were visiting their child'.

Algren (1985) studied 20 parents to discover not only the areas of care in which they participated but how much information they had been given by nurses regarding their role during their child's stay. Forty per cent of the parents were unsure as to whether they had been asked about this by staff and 60% said that they had 'definitely not' been consulted. Seventy per cent reported that nurses had not discussed the role that they might or should adopt while living-in on the ward and 30% felt that this had been vaguely alluded to. All of the parents in this study wished to participate in their child's care, especially again in areas such as changing, feeding and comforting as opposed to more technical and procedural tasks.

Stull and Deatrick (1986) used semi-structured interviews and encouraged parents to keep a diary in an attempt to discover 'more specific activities pertaining to parental involvement during a child's hospitalization'. Twenty-four parents of a handicapped child who had previous experience of being in hospital with the child described their activities during their stay. These were subsequently used as the basis for the construction of an instrument to measure parental participation (Deatrick *et al.,* 1986). It was found that the majority of parental activities were 'direct care activities' such as physical care and comforting. The researchers also identified as being important, areas of parental activity where parents were not directly involved in 'hands-on' care of their child. These were areas such as discussing the child with staff and spending time with other parents or alone.

The majority of studies regarding parent participation have focused on mothers. This is not surprising in view of the fact that it is usually mothers rather than fathers who stay in with their child during hospitalization although fathers have been playing a larger part in child-care in recent years. As part of a larger study, Knafl and Dixon (1984) surveyed 47 fathers whose children were in hospital to discover the nature of their participation in their child's care. Most fathers altered their routines, especially work, to enable them to visit the ward more often. The majority of the fathers (44) defined their role in the child's care in similar terms to mothers, that is, as being there primarily to provide emotional support, entertainment and comfort.

Most commonly the discourse on parental involvement and participation within the professional literature centres on parents as performers of tasks that they will perform in order to feel useful. Parents were expected to feel that they were being useful both to their child and to the hospital. Meadow (1969, p. 366) exemplified this understanding when he proposed that 'nurses must be trained in how to share care with a resident mother and how to use her as an efficient and willing source of labour'. Similarly, Hawthorne (1974, p. 133) noted that in one ward in her study, a visiting hours information slip stated that 'we would appreciate it if parents of younger children would visit at appropriate meal times in order to feed children when possible'.

Again, in a more recent study, Keane *et al.* (1986), rather than supporting the idea that all children and parents could benefit from being together during hospitalization, suggested a need to 'clarify the characteristics of mothers and children most likely to benefit from residential facilities', since these parents 'are users of resources' (p. 253, 247).

The literature on parent participation exemplifies a technological and instrumental understanding of the person (Taylor, 1985a; Benner, 1985b) which is ultimately objectifying and which may have helped to ensure that other ways of understanding parents' and nurses' experiences have been overlooked. Specifically, despite carrying out several manual and computerized literature searches during this study, I was unable to discover studies which had sought to understand the lived experience of resident parents' participation from a more phenomenological perspective.

A further omission in much of the literature on parent participation is that the situation within which participation occurs seems neglected in favour of isolating context-free variables. For example, studies that acknowledge the influence of nurses on parents' participation have focused on nurses' attitudes in relation to their place of work, level of education and rank (Seidl and Pilliterri, 1967; Seidl, 1969; Goodell, 1979; Gill, 1987a). Such studies addressed neither nurses' lived experiences of participating in care with resident parents nor the nature of their ongoing practices related to parental participation and involvement. There was also no attempt made to explore the meanings that the summary phrase 'parent participation' has for nurses. In order to see how previous researchers and writers have examined this wider situation, I now consider the nurse–parent relationship.

1.1.3 Nurses and live-in parents

While nurses welcomed many of the Platt Report's recommendations such as the need for children's nurses to have specialist paediatric training, they were less enthusiastic about parents having virtually unrestricted access to the wards. In short, they appeared wary of the idea of parents participating on any other than nurses' terms. This was made clear by one nurse who wrote that 'it is a fact that, in the enthusiasm for open house for mothers, many of the problems this can present to medical and nursing staff tend to be overlooked. They are, after all, professionals in their field, and having amateurs around is, as one suggested, like having wives on board ship' Anstice (1970, p. 1517).

The situation that developed in the post-Platt era could be described as one where the presence of parents was tolerated rather than actively encouraged and where parents were often resented and not positively valued. Early American studies pointed to parents being seen as 'a problem' for nurses (Moran, 1963; Mahaffy, 1964) and to the underlying and often open mutual resentment that existed between these two groups (Berman, 1966). A similar situation was reported in the UK by Brain and MacLay (1968) who carried out a controlled experiment in 'allowing' certain parents to live-in with their child during and after ENT surgery. At the end of the experiment the researchers noted of the nursing staff that 'they were unanimous in their opinion that they preferred the children to be admitted on their own' (p. 279).

The reasons given by the nurses were that they found it easier to carry out procedures when parents were not there, they were able to make more personal contact with the child in their parent's absence and that some mothers were 'difficult' (p. 297). In contrast to these findings, Hawthorne (1974, p. 125) noted that 84.5% of nurses interviewed for her study denied that mothers got in the way of nurses. However, she also found that only one of nine wards studied encouraged mothers to become resident.

This 'resistance at ward level to the admission of mothers or fathers' was also noted by Stacey *et al.* (1970, p. 151) in the first of the 'Swansea studies' into children in hospital. In a later, related study, Hall (1977, p. 178) noted that for nurses, 'parents too, were a feature of the ward that was disliked'. In the final part of this group of studies, Stacey (1979, p. 206) continued to find that 'parents tend still to be treated as outsiders and to be tolerated rather than integrated', while Hall (1979, p. 163) stated that 'one interesting feature to arise out of the questionnaires administered (. . .) was the strong negative view of parents held by some nurses.'

Paediatric nurses had a rich vocabulary of disparagement for parents. The 'thick' mother seemed not to understand what is happening, the 'neurotic' mother worried about her child, the 'lazy' mother did not help enough and the 'troublemaker' did not seem to fit in to the generally accepted mould of what a good live-in parent should be. Anstice (1970, p. 1517) was disarmingly blunt in her description of 'some mothers': 'Some are a support to the child and a help to the nurse. Some, fussy and neurotic, manage to be neither. Some again are unbelievably stupid, or perhaps it is too easy to forget that they just do not know things that any nurse takes for granted.'

Much of the research on parents in hospital, and particularly the 'Swansea studies', were characterized by several features. A pervasive sociological perspective led to the nurse–parent relationship being viewed through the lens of general sociological theory. Thus the parents' and nurses' experiences were filtered through theoretical screens of 'power and control', 'treatment and moral careers', 'ideologies' and Goffmanesque 'dramaturgy'. The results of such studies are no doubt of sociological interest. However, I suggest that what was ignored or filtered out is equally worthy of study. It is those meaningful and relational dimensions of the lived experiences of parents and nurses that I attempted to uncover in this study.

A second major characteristic of the surveyed literature is its focus on what Benner (1984, p. 219) calls 'deficit mode' thinking. This literature is almost uniformly critical of both nurses and hospitals. Nurses are cast in the role of agents of social control and parents seem no more than passive ciphers in an institutional conspiracy that seeks to control and oppress them (see, e.g., Beuf, 1979). The language of social structures and of given theories have been placed like a template over the study situation, occluding a vision of the everyday meanings, practices and understandings that are more local and contextual. To criticize such literature for exhibiting deficit mode thinking is not to suggest the existence of an idealized world where all professional practice is laudable and where all nurse–parent relationships are mutually successful and satisfying. It is rather to propose that certain theoretical frameworks and research approaches represent a search for detached theoretical knowledge that serves the interests of social engineering. While such perspectives seem all too ready to explain the social world, they are ill-equipped to recognize and describe aspects of both nurses' and parents' practices and experiences that may be more positive.

Pill (1970), for example, described an observational approach based upon a sociology of suspicion and a notion that a subject–object dichotomy is both inevitable and desirable. Within this approach, the researcher seemed merely a 'research tool', standing above, rather than beside, the participants and reporting on 'the facts of the situation'. Significantly here, Pill (1970, p. 88) expressed the need for not only a theoretical screen, but also a physical one: 'Ideally, of course a one-way screen or other device for concealment would have been desirable, but this is obviously impossible to arrange in the average ward.'

The attempt to understand nurse–parent relationships from this stance seems to have led to other oversights. For example, Pill (1970, p. 121) also remarked that 'in the nature of things, there are long stretches of time when the routine care has been done and the nurse is merely keeping an eye on things'. Such a comment betrays a misunderstanding of the complexity of nursing. It is also testimony to the value of later work by Benner (1984; 1989) and MacLeod (1990), among others, who have uncovered the wealth of nursing expertise and caring practices that can be so easily glossed over by summary phrases such as 'routine care' and 'merely keeping an eye on things'.

I suggest that the 'Swansea studies' can be better understood by considering their production within the sociological climate of the time. The late 1960s and 1970s were something of a 'golden age' for British sociology, highlighted by its expansion and popularity within Higher Education (Payne et al., 1981). Sociology became synonymous with the ability to uncover, expose and understand what was 'really happening' within society and its institutions. Sociological thinking was critical thinking, but with the emphasis firmly placed upon critical. It sought to radically critique, to unmask, to explain the world in terms of whichever theoretical perspective was employed. However, it seemed that such critical sociology, exemplified by the 'Swansea studies', lacked the reflectiveness necessary to turn its critical gaze inward. This was evidenced in Bell and Newby's (1977) discussion of the second 'Banbury Study' undertaken by Stacey et al. (1975). One of the research team, Bell, described how he felt constrained from writing what he believed to be a completely frank personal account of the research study. The strong impression given in this account is that if Bell was too critical, possible legal action might well have been initiated by other members of the research team (Bell and Newby, 1977, p. 170–173.).

Significantly, for a growing and expanding profession, sociology was also careful to ensure that problems were cast in sociological terms in order that solutions could also be similarly defined. From this perspective, the analysis and proposed solutions of Stacey et al. (1970) and Hall and Stacey (1979) seem rather self-serving. They claimed that the problems of children and their parents in hospital required a sociological understanding, which lead inevitably to their call for 'social scientists to be in interaction with doctors and nurses' (Stacey 1979, p. 208) and for increased teaching of social sciences throughout all nursing and medical education. Strong's comments are, I believe, particularly apposite in relation to the previous sociological studies of children in hospital: 'Scepticism has considerable dramatic rewards. In writing in this fashion, sociologists both formulate themselves as members of some insightful and incorruptible elite and, at the same time, gain considerable pleasure by the exposure and thus potential overthrow of those whom they dislike' (Strong, 1979b, p. 201).

Of particular relevance to the question of parents in paediatrics was a further body of predominantly qualitative research studies, undertaken by Hayes and Knox and Robinson and Thorne in Canada, which focused on children with a long-term chronic illness. Knox and Hayes (1983) and Hayes and Knox (1984) used a grounded theory approach to examine the experience of stress in 40 parents. It is unclear whether these parents were resident but Knox and Hayes (1983, p. 221) did note that mothers spent more time in hospital than fathers and 'felt a need to be present'.

These researchers hinted that parents experienced fundamental changes when they recalled those who spoke of their whole life changing and parents who described how no-one but another parent could really understand the nature of their experience. However, Hayes and Knox did not follow this ontological lead, preferring to develop an account of the parents' stress in terms of the discrepant perspectives that they argued existed between parents and health-care staff. They also used role theory to suggest that parents' stress experiences were related to changed perceptions of their role when their child was hospitalized.

These studies were important in focusing attention on the perspectives of parents of hospitalized children and highlighted several salient aspects of parents' experiences. I suggest however that the adopted perspectives of role theory and an essentially mechanistic view of stress based on the work of Selye (1976) and Scott *et al.* (1980), obscured much of the parents' personal meaning which these studies might have revealed. Role theory is premised on the dualistic assumption that our being is distinct from our social practices. From this basis it is perhaps inevitable that the meaning of being a parent in these studies came to be seen in terms of end-goals and the playing of a part with associated connotations of inauthenticity. The conclusions of these studies were not quite so trivializing however as Stacey *et al.*'s (1970, p. 151) view, that parents were unable to 'play the role of "mother-in-the-ward"'.

I argue later that a parent's way of being-in-the-world (Heidegger, 1962) cannot be adequately captured in the objective language of roles that suggests chosen ends rather than integrated sets of practices through which we interpret and understand ourselves and order our everyday activities (Dreyfus, 1983). A further limitation of Hayes and Knox's role perspective is that it concentrates upon only one group of 'actors', the parents, thus losing the sense of shared human being which marks out our everyday experience. The 'role' of parent of a hospitalized child makes little sense in isolation from, say, the role of the paediatric nurse due to the importance of shared understandings and common meanings.

It is difficult to evaluate the contribution made by Selye's and Scott *et al.*'s stress theory to these studies. Although they were described as 'central to the background of the study' (Hayes and Knox, 1984, p. 344), in the theoretical framework section, they were not mentioned again in this paper. A concluding question raised by Hayes and Knox (1984, p. 340) was 'What is the nature of the nurse–parent relationship in hospital?' This is one of the questions which this book addresses.

The research of Robinson and Thorne (1984) was also significant in relation to nurse–parent relationships in paediatrics. As part of the 'Health Care Relationships Project', qualitative interviews were carried out with families with an adult member who had cancer and families with a chronically ill child. Robinson and Thorne contended that relationships between health-care professionals, patients and parents developed according to discernible, predictable stages. These were 'Naive Trusting', 'Disenchantment' and 'Guarded Alliance'. As their titles suggested, these stages were characterized by families' increasing disenchantment with the nature of their relationships with health care providers until the stage of 'Guarded Alliance' was reached. This stage was achieved when the parents and patients were more aware of professionals' limitations and where their trust was reconstructed on the basis of a more active and informed stance (Robinson and Thorne, 1984, p. 599–600).

A major difficulty in assessing the plausibility of Robinson and Thorne's thesis is that the study and interpretive conclusions were presented with almost no supporting evidence in the form of interview data. While the researchers' thinking and ideas were well represented, the voices and accounts of the study participants remained largely unheard. The progression from 'Naive Trusting' to 'Guarded Alliance' seemed seductively reassuring. It suggested a forward-moving, linear development that sits comfortably with Western and traditional scientific under-standing. While the researchers cannot be held responsible for how other nurses may use this model of relationship development, there is a danger that nurses may seize on these labels of progression in order to designate rather than understand parents' lived experiences. For example, I remember being able to recite James Robertson's stages of a child's 'settling-in' to hospital, Elizabeth Kubler-Ross's stages of dying, the four stages of group formation and the stages of the nursing process. How great an insight or understanding these stages afforded is debatable. I suspect that what was achieved by this thinking in stages was in truth a distanc-ing from the person and their lived experiences, for they were now at least partially hidden by a label.

A further difficulty in evaluating Robinson and Thorne's work is that there seemed to be some confusion as to the theoretical basis and research method used in the studies. In the original report of the 'Health Care Relationships Project', the researchers stated only that their theory was based on 'separate qualitative studies' (Robinson and Thorne, 1984, p. 599). In a later study, Thorne and Robinson (1988a, p. 783) stated that: 'analysis relied upon the grounded theory method of qualitative research (Glaser and Strauss, 1967) and resulted in the confirmation of a three-stage process of relationship evolution (Thorne and Robinson, in press). However a different account of their theoretical approach was offered in the 'in press' paper to which they referred. In this report, Thorne and Robinson (1988b, p. 295) claimed that: 'the phenomenological paradigm of qualitative methodology directed both the process of constructing accounts with informant family members and analysis of the data that emerged'.

This seeming contradiction indicates either a confusion as to the nature of grounded theory and phenomenology or an assumption that the two terms are somehow interchangeable.

1.1.4 Parents' accounts

A further body of writing reviewed was parents' accounts of their experiences of visiting or living-in with their child. Within the research approach of this study, these accounts are not viewed as being merely anecdotal, private or sub-jective. In the collection of solicited parents' letters compiled by Robertson (1962), parents described how much they valued being able to stay with their sick child and, alternatively, how distressing it was for parents who were forbidden from doing this. Significant in these parents' letters was how grateful they were for what they believed was the 'privilege' of being allowed to live-in and how they seemed prepared to tolerate almost any level of inconvenience and discomfort to this end.

Parents' feelings of disorientation, disordered time perception and 'unreality' during living-in were described by Turner (1984), Hilton (1982) and Beckett (1986). Many parents described intense feelings of guilt, anger, depression and physical exhaustion at various points during their living-in (Nolan, 1981; Turner,

1984; Hilton, 1982; Beckett, 1986; Smith, 1987). In their relations with hospital staff, parents described a gamut of emotions and involvement. Feelings of helplessness and uncertainty were described by Turner (1984) and Smith (1987) while Anonymous (1984) and Arango (1990) wrote of their feelings of being excluded from discussion and information about their child and of having no-one who genuinely understood their experience and needs. Webb (1977), Turner (1984) and Martin (1986) explained that they found everyday child care tasks strange and difficult to perform within the ward. Some of these parents described their relationships with nurses, highlighting the value that they attached to nurses who were open, honest, informal, caring and willing to listen and talk, (Khoo, 1972; Turner, 1984; Martin, 1986; Beckett, 1986; Smith, 1987). However, parents also described encounters with staff whom they felt had been rude, abrupt, arrogant and unhelpful (Robertson, 1962; Webb, 1977; Hilton, 1982; Turner, 1984; Smith, 1987).

The purpose of reviewing parents' accounts was to gain an initial understanding of their perspective of living-in and of the ways in which they described their experiences. These parents' accounts provided potentially valuable insights and sensitizing ideas which were further explored within this study.

1.2 SUMMARY AND CONCLUSIONS

This chapter has focused on four bodies of literature concerning: the historical development of current paediatric care philosophy; parental participation and involvement in their child's care; resident or live-in parents; and parents' own accounts of their experiences.

The historical development of paediatrics saw parents' expertise and knowledge of their child usurped by professionals. This related not only to the child's physical care but also to what has become known as their emotional and psychological care. Ostensibly, the Platt Report was an attempt to counter this movement by advocating a greater sensitivity towards parent–child separation and greater parental involvement. However, the slow and patchy implementation of the Platt Report's recommendations, especially in relation to parental living-in and involvement, pointed to the considerable oversights which flawed the report. While the lack of a wider sociological perspective may have contributed to lack of progress in 'humanizing' paediatric care, such a perspective alone offers only a limited understanding of the lived experiences and meanings of resident parents and paediatric nurses.

The literature on parental involvement was notable for its basis in an instrumental and technological understanding of parents as being essentially of functional value. From this perspective, parents too readily became problems to be managed or resources to be more effectively used by ward staff. This literature also seemed content to leave the fundamental meaning of parent participation unexplored and unproblematic while opting to measure and propose socially engineered solutions.

Studies that have sought to explain the nurse–parent relationship tended to cloak the participants' personal and shared meanings in sociological concepts. The legitimacy of these labels was made difficult to appraise due to the researchers' common practice of assigning them while offering the reader minimal supporting data, in the form of participants' accounts.

Parents' own accounts offered interesting insights, but most of those published were brief and tended to concentrate on the more dramatic emotions and events which parents experienced. These accounts often overlooked the meanings related to the more everyday nature of the parents' lived experience and the practices that sustained this.

This review has shown that the lived experiences of parents and nurses have been largely overlooked in previous research. This has resulted in significant gaps in our understanding of how parents experience staying with their child in hospital and how parents' relationships with paediatric nurses develop. If paediatric nursing is to continue to advocate and develop a philosophy of care based upon mutuality and partnership with parents, then nurses need a deeper understanding of the nature of parents' experiences and how these relate to their own nursing practices.

An alternative to an instrumental understanding of parents and nurses is to consider the person as constituted by a web of relationships with others (Dreyfus, 1983; Bellah *et al.*, 1985; Taylor, 1985a). In this way the relational and contextual aspects of lived experiences and relationships may be uncovered and the voices of the research participants may be heard throughout the study. If this is achieved, then readers will be in a better position to appraise the interpretations offered. Finally, there seemed a need for a research approach to these experiences that was not linear and progressive but essentially phenomenological, hermeneutic, and dialogical (Bleicher, 1980; Benner, 1985a; Taylor, 1985b) where 'the aim is not to uncover universals or laws but rather to explicate context and world' (Rabinow and Sullivan, 1979, p. 13).

I now begin this 'uncovering' by describing what was involved for parents as they learned to 'parent in public'.

Becoming a live-in parent: 'parenting in public'

2.1 INTRODUCTION

In this chapter I describe how the parents experienced their situation during the early part of their stay in the ward and how their way of being a parent began to change in response to the different situation in which they now found themselves.

The reasons which parents gave for deciding to live-in will be presented and discussed as these were illustrative of several issues. While some parents had very little idea of what to expect, others had particular expectations and preconceptions of what would be involved in living-in. Several other factors helped to influence parents' early days in the ward. Not surprisingly, the nature of the child's illness or injury was a factor here and this is discussed in relation to the process of admission to the ward, drawing out both contrasts and similarities from different parents' experiences.

Interpretation of the parents' accounts suggested that two related aspects of being a live-in parent were particularly important at this time. Parents now had to be parents within a unique and very different social situation at a time when they were under great stress and extremely afraid. Secondly, this experience could affect, in the Heideggerian sense, parents' being-in-the-world in terms of their concerns, understandings and practices. Here I examine the meaning of these changes in relation to particular aspects of the parents' early days on the ward.

Uncertainty and confusion characterized this early period. Parents were uncertain regarding what they could and could not do with and for their child. They seemed, however, to experience a deeper uncertainty that could call into question a parent's more fundamental sense of being and worth. The various ways in which parents tried to adapt to this new situation will be described.

Parents were entering a situation where, possibly for the first time, they were being expected to devolve some of their autonomy over their child and his or her care. They may have found themselves negotiating permission to participate, not only in the more 'technical' aspects of the child's care but in what may previously have been seen as the some of the most basic areas of their child's care.

The context of the ward was an influential factor during the parent's stay. This was a strange new setting in which to live with your child. The setting was certainly strange physically and geographically but it was also a situation that acted directly upon previously routine and unproblematic areas of child care and being a parent. The simplest and most taken-for-granted child-care practices were distorted in their rhythm and often in their meaning for parents. A particularly illuminating example of how the context of the ward influenced the parents' normal child-care practice was the issue of disciplining the hospitalized child. Live-in parents' understandings of this issue are therefore explored.

Finally, I draw upon the accounts of the nurses in order to examine how their perspectives and practices affected parents at this time. In particular I will discuss how nurses formed their initial assessments and impressions of live-in parents and how, within the context of the ward, the concept of family and parental identity come to be created, both morally and socially.

2.1.1 Parents' reasons for wishing to live-in

In the interviews with the parents, I asked how their child had come to be admitted to hospital and to explain why they had decided to live-in. The parents' accounts revealed several reasons for making this choice.

(a) Circumstantial reasons

Circumstantial reasons related primarily to the distance away from the hospital that parents lived. In such circumstances, additional to the inconvenience of travelling long distances was the cost of daily return travel that could have been prohibitive. One mother who had already spent several weeks in the ward explained that

> Well, more or less because it's too far to travel, it's costing too much to come in and out (. . .) we've worked it out that, by the time we get taxis and trains and buses, it's working out at roughly £10 . . . that's coming here and going back. (15, p. 1)

(b) Instrumental reasons

Instrumental reasons related to more specifically functional parental concerns. Here parents described how they wanted to live-in in order to help their child in tangible or practical ways, for example by helping with their child's daily care or by being available if consent forms had to be signed. As one mother explained:

> We wanted to do jobs instead of just sitting there (. . .) so that we felt as if we were helping. (5, p. 3)

Three of the mothers had to live-in as they were breast feeding. One of these mothers explained the importance of her presence:

My wee boy's just 8 weeks and I'm breast feeding him so it was really important that I stay in (. . .) but even if I wasn't breast feeding him, I'd still be there, 'cos – just for the bonding, really. . . . (28, Mother 2, p. 4)

Parents also described how their living-in would be 'a help to the nurses' as they were 'so busy'. This is an issue that is taken up in more detail in Chapter 4. As one mother explained:

You see, I think if I'm here that's one less for the nurse to look after. (28, Mother 1, p. 6)

(c) Protective and advocacy reasons

Protective or advocacy reasons were given by mothers who felt that they had to be with their child in the ward in order to protect them from what they saw as some of the possible ill effects of hospitalization. Parents were, for example, very aware of other children in the ward, especially young babies, and would comment if they had been 'left to cry' for long periods. This was taken as a sign that either that nurses didn't really care about distressed children or that they were too busy to give them the attention that they desired. The parents' presence therefore became insurance against their child being similarly neglected. These mothers explained that

. . . like, I wouldn't leave him in here anyway 'cos the nurses would just leave him to greet [weep] and cry. (26, Mother 4, p. 2)

. . . at the weekend they [the nurses] were really rushing about and you see various children around the ward crying for something and there just **aren't** the nurses to cope with that sort of demand (. . .) and you think, well if I wasn't here and my child started whimpering about something, or just wanted to go to the toilet or something . . . would there be someone to deal with it? . . . and you think **I've got to be there**. (27, Mother 1, p. 56)

Watching and listening to other children crying in the ward distressed the mothers. One described how 'it tears at a mother's stomach to hear a child crying' (27, p. 32), yet parents felt that it would have been inappropriate to go and comfort someone else's child unless this had been arranged with the parents beforehand.

(d) Emotional and supportive reasons

Parents also described emotional and supportive reasons for living-in with their child. These had a predominantly negative emphasis, where parents would describe how, in their absence, the child would possibly suffer some emotional or psychological upset as a result of the hospitalization. They also spoke of hospital as being traumatic enough for the child without the added trauma that they felt their absence would entail. The mother of a four-year-old girl due to undergo plastic surgery described this:

> Well, Jenny is the type of girl, she's a mummy's girl, I can't go anywhere without her and I thought if, here, the thought of going into hospital alone . . . I thought, no, I have to stay with her. I was frightened of how she would feel with the fear. (14, p. 1)

This mother's comment suggested that parents' reasons for wishing to stay with the child concerned not only the child's emotional well-being but the parent's also. Another mother and father described this when they explained that by living-in, they believed that they would be helping not only their daughter, but themselves. They explained that they were

> . . . helping Mary and through her we were helping ourselves as well you know. (5, p. 3)

Other parents had more positive reasons for living-in. A mother whose nine-year-old son had undergone several hospitalizations for repair of a hypospadias described how her presence had a beneficial effect on her son's emotional state. Because she was there, he would be less likely to be shy and reticent during his stay and therefore be less likely to be overlooked in the general 'busyness' of the ward.

> 'Cos I'm here he's a different kid, but if I wasn't here, and there was something wrong with him, I don't know so much now but even a year ago, he'd have just laid there and not said anything, he wouldn't have complained . . . and I think that was one of the reasons I wouldn't have liked not to have been here, plus if he was bored he'd have just lain there and not made a fuss, that other kids would have made to get attention . . . which is quite hard to believe when you see him (laughs). . . . (13, p. 14)

2.1.2 Deciding to live-in

Typically, parents seemed not to have deliberated at length over their decision to live-in. They described this as an automatic, almost reflex action and not a decision where they had carefully considered possible advantages and disadvantages. For these parents, not living-in with their child was simply not an option to be considered. This was evident in the accounts of several parents:

> I didn't realize that she was so ill, we thought she only had gastroenteritis, they didn't realize that she had haemolytic uraemic syndrome . . . and then you're in an ambulance and here's lights flashing, doctors at the Sick Kids waiting for this child at the door . . . nope . . . it didn't dawn on me to do anything else, bar stay. (27, Mother 4, p. 3)

When a child was admitted as an emergency, this would often positively influence the parent's decision to live-in. One mother explained how this situation rendered living-in as being the only possible course of action for her:

> We had no choice, because the baby's so ill. . . . I just couldn't leave him, basically . . . in fact I don't know what I would have done if they'd said to me that I couldn't . . . it just wasn't a consideration not to stay. (17, p. 1)

Another mother felt that her decision was equally automatic:

> I just automatically said, 'I'm staying with her', I just never sort of thought of anything else. (10, p. 14)

Parents of children who had been admitted from waiting lists for elective surgery often felt equally strongly that living-in was not an option but an essential course of action where they had no real choice or desire to do other than stay with their child. One such mother described this:

> No. No, I never gave it any thought, it was just automatic I'd be there, and that was it . . . and that was why I spent the first two nights by her bed, so that I was there, till she sort of got used to the fact that she was in hospital and Mummy was staying. (. . .) In my mind I was going to be with her no matter what. (14, p. 2)

Parents did not seem to anticipate difficulties involved in living-in and seemed genuinely surprised when I mentioned to them that living-in was a relatively new aspect of paediatric hospitalization. At this, one mother said flatly that if she had not been allowed to stay, then she would have discharged her child from the hospital immediately.

A recurrent feature of parents' explanations was the strength of feeling that accompanied their responses. It was clear that parents saw living-in not so much as a detached or rational decision that was to be weighed up and considered but as a strongly emotional response, rooted in parents' clear sense of their being as parents. This primordial relationship between parent and child was well described by the following mother's comments:

> But you don't give birth to a baby just to leave it, I mean, if you've got a baby who's only 10 weeks old, I mean, he's new to the world, you don't have him to leave him when he's ill. (26, Mother 5, p. 4)

This intensity of relationship between parent and child was heightened when the child was threatened by illness, disease or injury. Two mothers described how living-in with their child in hospital was not simply a continuation of what was expected of them as parents, but was in fact a heightened expectation, at a time when their child needed them more than ever:

> I think because I knew she was in pain and she was frightened, and I think that I felt that if I went away and deserted her, that it would make it worse

'cos she just wouldn't understand why Mummy had went away. I mean if she's ever fallen and grazed herself or banged her head you automatically are there and pick them up and I mean, if I went away when she was in the worst pain she's ever had and sort of deserted her, I mean . . . it would be cruel. (10, p. 14)

I'm normally with her anyway 24 hours, most of the day, and this being an extremely traumatic experience for her, then it's more important still to be with her. (26, Mother 1, p. 1)

While parents offered particular reasons for deciding to live-in initially, their experiences within the ward could alter their justification for both the initial decision and their continued stay. This was most apparent in the accounts of parents who described an incident or example of what they considered to be poor care. When this occurred parents were more likely to view their role as live-in parents as being increasingly that of the child's protector.

This was vividly described by a mother of a baby who had undergone surgery to repair a pilonidal sinus. On one occasion her baby's dressing was being renewed by two relatively junior student nurses or 'wee school lassies' as she described them. This mother and her husband stood in the treatment room, distressed, enraged and almost in tears, while they watched an extremely painful and unpleasant procedure being performed by nurses who, the mother felt, 'didn't have a clue'. This was the most traumatic part of the parents' stay in hospital and after this incident she felt very strongly that

after experiencing what we experienced, both of us there [her and her husband], having to witness our child being put through a helluva lot of pain unnecessarily . . . I don't think that I would **ever, ever**, leave him again, or any of my children in a hospital again, after witnessing that. (26, Mother 5, p. 58)

Parents' reasons for deciding to live-in suggested that they had certain expectations of what their role might be while living-in. Instrumental reasons indicated that parents expected to play some active part in their hospitalized child's care. Implicit within emotional and supportive reasons was the expectation that parents would play a part in making traumatic aspects of hospitalization less so for their child, perhaps by being with them at particularly difficult times such as during an injection or before a general anaesthetic. Although parental reasons for wishing to live-in have been described individually here, they were neither mutually exclusive nor even clearly separable. It was common for parents to describe, for example, both instrumental and emotional and supportive reasons as part of a wider awareness of the totality of their child's needs.

However, to consider parents' decisions as being essentially rational and calculated would, I argue, be to misunderstand the essence of the parents' desire to be with their child at this time. For parents, this was a time of fear, anguish and uncertainty where rational thinking was often quite impossible. Understanding how parents felt at this time suggests that their decision to live-in was no rational decision at all. As Benner and Wrubel (1989) observe:

> For one who is fully committed to the situation, as a parent might be to a sick child, questions about abandoning the child or leaving the situation simply do not show up as options. The parent does not feel 'brave' or courageous for staying in the situation because there is just no other way to be. The parent has a world-defining relationship with the child that does not allow for even imagining a life without the child. (Benner and Wrubel, 1989, p. 82)

The accounts of the parents supported this view. Leaving or abandoning their child was not accorded the status of an option for parents. At this most threatening and traumatic time for their child, they needed to be with them in every sense possible.

2.1.3 Admission: becoming 'a different parent'

Towards the beginning of the interviews with parents I asked them to describe their child's admission and their first few days of living-in. This was intended to offer an opening for discussion which parents would find relatively easy and also to gain a more detailed insight into parents' perceptions of their transition from being a parent at home to being a parent within a paediatric ward.

Understandably, parents described the strangeness of the new situation that they had entered, not only in relation to the physical environment but also in relation to the organizational rhythms and practices with which they were now expected to comply. This section explores the nature of this strangeness for parents and the influences that helped to shape it.

Parents' entry into the situation began prior to being admitted with their child. Admission to hospital was a part of the whole process of the child's illness or injury, not a discrete event performed at an isolated point in time. How parents perceived the introduction to the ward and the initial part of their stay in hospital was influenced by several factors. The nature and meaning of the child's illness or injury for the parent was important in this respect. Where the child had been admitted as an emergency, this seemed to have had a more traumatic effect upon the parents' perceptions of their first days in the ward. One mother whose child had been scalded at home described how her child's extensive bandaging and the entire ward environment seemed to conspire against her, constantly accuse her and fuel her feelings of guilt:

> Terrible. It was like you were never away from what happened, everything was going through your head . . . you kept blaming yourself and couldn't sleep . . . horrible. (25, Mother 2, p. 5)

Another mother whose baby had been transferred to one of the hospital's intensive care areas described the initially disorienting effect that the severity of her baby's illness had upon herself and her husband:

> Every day was just the same, days and nights just sort of merged into one and it was just so traumatic, just because of [his] condition, I mean nights were turned into days 'cos we were just up all the time 'cos he was on a knife edge basically, he could have died at any moment, so we sort of . . . we went up to our room in the Mothers' Unit, dozed for a couple of hours, but basically we were always there, we were always either in the ICU or in the corridor. We were never anywhere else apart from to eat. (17, p. 4)

This disruption contrasted with mothers who had known in advance that their child was coming into hospital for a planned admission and whose children were not seen by either staff or parents as being seriously ill. One mother whose daughter was due to have a comparatively small skin graft, explained that although she had found her first few days to be 'strained', her admission to the ward had not been characterized by the trauma described by others. She explained:

> Well, we came in on the Sunday night after tea and that was fine, quite relaxed, it wasn't a busy ward, she was a bit excited, she had her toilet bag and new slippers, you know . . . the novelty of going up and down the ward, she was fine. (14, p. 2–3)

However, the fact that the child's admission was planned did not eradicate all parental anxieties. For parents who had previous experience of being in hospital with their child, these memories could form the basis of current anxieties. The parents of a child who was having further surgery to repair a cleft lip and palate defect described the fears accompanying the technology that was so familiar to hospital staff:

> **PD:** Can you remember how you felt, at the beginning, the first week?
> **Father:** Terrified.
> **Mother:** We were both frightened.
> **PD:** Can you remember what about?
> **Mother:** In case it was the same as the last time . . . she had everything attached to her when she came back from theatre . . . she had an oxygen box over her head the last time and she had the drip on, naturally, and she had a heart monitor as well . . . there just seemed to be leads everywhere. (12, p. 7–8)

Parents soon realized that being a parent in hospital would not be a simple continuation of being a parent at home. The nature and meaning of their parenting practices undertaken in the ward changed within this new context. What could also change was their sense of self and being as a parent. One parent expressed this very clearly, saying:

> It's not like being the same parent is it? . . . You're like a different parent. (27, Mother 3, p. 9)

This perception of the unreality of their situation was expressed by other parents who spoke of their feelings of being 'in a dream' during this early stage of their living-in. I suggest that one important factor that influenced this change was the uncertainty that they experienced. Parents at home are recognized as being 'the experts' in matters concerning their child and indeed professionals often claim to defer to and respect parents' intimate knowledge of their child (Strong, 1979a). Yet in the parents' accounts, they typically spoke of being uncertain, uninformed and confused. This was an uncertainty that seemed to permeate every aspect of their living-in. Uncertainty surrounded their understanding of their child's condition and treatment, their role as live-in parents, the finding out of information and their very being as parents. I now consider this parental uncertainty more closely.

2.1.4 Parental uncertainty: the 'emotional roller-coaster'

Parents described how feelings of uncertainty began to form shortly after admission when they found themselves in the position of no longer being the 'experts' in matters concerning their child. They now had to discover information from others regarding their child's treatment, progress and prognosis. Parents described how their early days in the ward were characterized by attempts to adapt their ways of being a parent in order to adjust to and to better understand their new situated being and its demands. I use the term 'situation' in its wider Heideggerian sense (Heidegger, 1962), to refer not simply to a physical environment but to a world that encompasses temporality, concerns, constraints, issues and information.

From the initial conversations and interviews with the parents it was clear that finding out information and developing an understanding of the situation was of great importance. Interpretation of the initial interviews and of later more focused interviews created several codes related to larger themes of 'uncertainty' and 'finding out'.

Parents' sense of uncertainty seemed to relate most often to the child's treatment and prognosis. For example, nurses spoke of how difficult it was to give any definite information regarding the child's prognosis to parents of a child who had sustained a severe head injury or a scald. The trajectory and ultimate prognosis for such children could be quite different and difficult to state precisely during the early stages.

The anxieties resulting from the ward's unfamiliarity and from uncertainty were described by one mother as being in striking contrast to her familiar routine at home:

When you come home and do the washing and ironing . . . I'd much rather be doing that, this is a different, this is a mental strain, not a physical strain I think in here, 'cos you're living on your nerves all the time, you know, wondering what's happening, what's going on. (2, p. 34)

The anxiety created by uncertainty was among the most distressing aspects of their stay in hospital. Several mothers described this:

> Not knowing, that's the worst of everything, as I've said, no-one can answer any questions you ask. (4, p. 9)

> The uncertainty is the worst thing of all. It's actually worse than anything. (5, p. 43)

> It was this not knowing that keeps you totally on tenterhooks the whole time and makes you very . . . very worried, you know. (9, p. 12)

Uncertainty seemed to hamper parents' ability to participate in their child's care as they felt unable to make the appropriate contributions, being unsure as to what these might be. One mother's description suggested this when she spoke of how her daughter was transferred from the more highly structured and organized environment of the cardiac surgery unit into a general surgical ward:

> . . . but then, after she got well enough not to need that special care . . . really it all appears to be confusion and I never know . . . I often have questions to ask, like where can I find a towel or will I give my child a bath, or did I ought to worry that she's itching under her plaster, you know . . . little things that probably aren't important, but I don't know whether they are or not. (26, Mother 1, p. 43)

Parents typically did not ascribe uncertainty to the fact that doctors and nurses were themselves genuinely unsure and uncertain (cf. Davis, 1963; Melia, 1987). Rather, parents believed that they were withholding knowledge and information. One mother used a telling medical metaphor as she described this process of being 'drip-fed' information:

> They don't seem to . . . I don't know if it's just me, like, but to me they seem to be holding back, you know, they only tell you so much and then somebody else will come in and they'll tell you a wee bit more information . . . so at the end of the day, you're getting most of the information but you're having to wait until maybe four or five or six different people give you all their wee bits. (5, p. 14)

A young mother felt that this holding back of information was being done to protect her because of her age:

> I found it quite difficult 'cos I don't think they're wanting to tell me too much and get me worried with me being so young. (15, p. 13)

Another mother, who was herself a nurse, acknowledged that doctors could not always give precise information but felt that this should not have meant that no useful information was forthcoming:

> I mean you don't actually want someone to come up and say 'in two hours time we'll do this' and 'in so many hours we'll do this', just, 'We hope that

this will happen,' or 'Probably this might happen,' but when you've **absolutely** no idea what's going on, it's really awful. (10, p. 51)

Some parents believed that information was being withheld in order to spare them undue anxiety or distress. However when parents lacked such information concerning their child's diagnosis, treatment or prognosis, it seemed that they were unable to establish any meaningful time frame to help them understand and manage the hospitalization. A mother whose child was recovering from a serious head injury tried to explain how she was monitoring her son's progress according to 'the charts' kept by his bed:

> There's nobody I have spoke to or read anything that has actually said, yes he had pressure on the brain, his right side was slow, and the doctors didn't know, but now this is wrong, you can't say to yourself, 'that's what's going to happen to him'. It gives you no idea of what could happen. (. . .) It says on the chart that he's still at two and needs to go to one. . . . Will it be next week or next month or will it be a year?. . . I don't know . . . there's no time limit for anything . . . there's no way they can say anything (. . .) I don't know what he's going into . . . just the same old answers . . . the favourite word here, **time** – time will tell. (4, p. 36, 43)

A father whose son had received extensive scalds and who had initially been in the burns unit's intensive care area, could not seem to relate to the spatial and temporal metaphors which doctors used to describe his son's condition. He described this confusion and uncertainty regarding the meaning of information: I used to see Dr Grey and would say, 'How is he?' and he'd say,

> 'Stable, but he's got a long way to go' and I would think, what does he mean by a long way to go? . . . A long way to go before he gets out the critical stage or a long way before he gets out?. . . this was confusing me and they're all still saying that, you know, what do they mean? . . . that he can get out in three weeks? (18, p. 33)

Parents' concentration upon longer-term issues was apparent particularly where the child's illness or injury had more obvious long-term implications. For example, the parents of the children who had sustained severe head injuries wanted to know about long-term prognosis while parents of children who had been burned or scalded wanted to discuss the extent of any future scarring. For nurses, these were questions that were shrouded in uncertainty and which they felt both unable and unqualified to answer. Nurses therefore tended to set the agenda for discussions with parents by confining themselves to more immediate issues.

Uncertainty also affected parents' abilities to prepare both themselves and their child for any treatments that were required. This preparation was seen by parents as being one of the main reasons for their living-in and was an area where they believed that they could make a unique contribution to the child's acceptance of treatments or procedures. When treatment schedules were changed without consultation with parents, or at short notice and with little or no explanation, parents felt themselves powerless and unable to 'psyche themselves up' in such a way as to manage the situation in more positive ways. This was a problem that seemed to particularly affect staff and parents in the burns unit. Resident parents here often explained that they were never sure whether their child would require skin grafting or how extensive such grafting might need to be. Staff described the difficulties that they faced in predicting such outcomes precisely and suggested to parents that a policy of 'wait and see' regarding the condition of the skin at each dressing change was best.

While parents usually accepted this as being reasonable, they were less tolerant of changes in treatment that they felt were the result of indecision or lack of competence. A mother whose daughter had scalded her legs and feet described how her daughter's proposed visits to theatre for dressing changes and possible skin grafting were changed repeatedly and for reasons that she could neither understand nor accept:

> I was told on Wednesday morning . . . they said, 'No we're **almost positive** she doesn't need a graft, and we're just going to take the dressing down again in the ward on the Thursday', so fine . . . then on Wednesday they come and say, 'She's going back to theatre on Friday'. So, Thursday morning I sign a consent form to say she's going to have a change of dressing in theatre on Friday morning. On Thursday afternoon that consent form is ripped up and another one is written saying she might need a skin graft on Friday morning . . . (laughs) . . . so she goes to theatre on Friday morning and comes back again without a skin graft . . . but they have decided by then that she will need one on the Monday but they couldn't do it on the Friday . . . by which time I was just about . . . I thought **I wish you lot would get your act together** and just finally decide. It was the feeling that I was being mucked about, if they'd said she needed one that was fine, I would have been prepared for it but . . . you were starting to feel elated and I'd been led to believe that if they changed the dressing and it was healed then I would get home that weekend, that's the way they were talking after the initial sort of theatre dressing. (10, p. 48–49)

The uncertainty and confusion experienced by this parent related not only to her resultant inability to be prepared for the skin graft, but also to the idea that the graft represented a setback in the child's treatment that she believed might not have been necessary.

It was important for parents to feel prepared. This was for more immediate events such as treatment and for the longer-term concerns regarding how they were going to function in the future as a family when the child was discharged. This was clearly more of a concern where the child's condition was going to require further or continuing attention at home. A mother described this in relation to the future of her daughter who had sustained a serious head injury:

If she will be disabled and handicapped, why can they not tell us so we can
... know what to expect in the future? I mean, we thought that being in a
coma she was sleeping, she'd come out of this and waken up and say, 'Oh,
Mummy, what's happened?' (5, p. 22)

Parents' uncertainty was also heightened by what they perceived to be conflicting information given by hospital staff. This often concerned the various rules
that some staff expected parents to adhere to. Several parents mentioned the ward
kitchen as being a particular source of conflict here. One mother explained:

I think the nurses are a little bit inconsistent themselves, for example, that
nurse said to you [another mother in the group], you're not supposed to eat
beside the bed but I'll turn a blind eye ... well, when I arrived in Ward X,
a nice nurse said to me, 'This is the kitchen, you're not supposed to use it,
but nobody will mind if you go and make a cup of coffee', and then a
little later, I didn't actually make a cup of coffee but I was in making a drink
for my little girl to save the nurses from doing it ... and one of the nurses
came in and said, 'Hrrrrrummmph! This kitchen isn't for public use!' ...
(laughs) ... so .... (26, Mother 1, p. 19–20)

This inconsistency on the part of some staff was often apparent to parents who,
as a result, felt that there were different rules for different parents. As one mother
noted:

... perhaps they make the rules to suit what parents they've got in at the
time. (26, Mother 5, p. 20)

This observation was partly borne out by my observations, that, especially in
relation to access to ward kitchens, parents who had lived-in for a sufficient
length of time and had become trusted, could eventually be granted permission
to use this area.

Conflicting advice and information given by nurses could lead parents to incur
the censure of one of the advising parties. A father and mother described such a
situation when he and his wife had been told that it would be in order for their
toddler to walk around the ward without wearing arm restraint splints:

Father: There was one thing happened the other day that I was about to get
awfully annoyed about ... one [nurse] had said she could walk about without her splints on, providing that either I was there or her mother was there
... so she was walking about literally the whole day, till the sisters changed
... the next sister comes along and says, 'That's not on, there's no way that
can happen!'
Mother: Mr Black [the consultant] is very strict about the splints being on
for a constant three weeks. ... I says, 'We wouldn't have taken it on ourselves to take them off, we were told to', so the staff nurse got a rollicking
for that.
Father: You see, what's happening is that one nurse is telling you one

thing, and another is telling you different . . . another nurse, who's maybe a bit more severe, she's telling you what she thinks (. . .) we just got a wee bit confused, you know. (12, p. 5–7)

In this example, the father saw this conflicting advice as being the result of nurses' individual personalities and of their degree of personal severity. He did not seem to consider this as being a confusion caused by a rule that was neither clear nor universally adhered to. Despite his initial anger at the episode, which was due in the main to the 'awfully abrupt' way that his wife had been reprimanded, there was an almost passive acceptance that he and his wife shared the responsibility for 'getting a wee bit confused'.

Being uncertain meant being afraid, anxious, lost, unconnected and powerless. This was well described by the parents of a girl who was comatose as a result of a head injury and who had developed a serious infection while in the ward that had caused her condition to deteriorate rapidly. She was transferred from the paediatric hospital to a nearby specialist head injury unit. For the illustrative vividness of its expression, her parents' account of this event is worth citing at length:

> **Mother:** They gave her an ECG CAP scan [*sic*], nothing showed up on the CAP scan, so they, the doctor says to me, 'There's nothing we can do for her, Mrs Pink, it's up to her now', so we thought she was going to die. . . . We phoned up all the family and told them she's not got long to live, it's up to the bairn now, they can't do anything for her . . . then they brought her back here [to the paediatric hospital] and rushed her into the intensive care unit, they're standing by with life support, they had her on a heart monitor, a breathing monitor, they had plugs on her head and every time you asked them something . . . 'Oh, it's just a matter of time, Mrs Pink.' (. . .) She had an arrest and they had to start her heart again (. . .) and then they found she had shigella and they gave her all the antibiotics under the sun (. . .) but the doctor's saying to you, 'We're very sorry, Mrs Pink, there's nothing we can do, it's up to her,' . . . and then thinking, well, the bairn's going to die because she's deteriorating . . . and then we get a row for thinking like that . . . (mother mimics a cheerful voice) 'She's not going to die, there's nothing wrong with her!' . . . **Jesus!** what are you supposed to think? (. . .) They try to hide it off you. (. . .) Now, every time we were coming in she was getting worse, I says, 'Well,' to my husband, 'do you think . . . she'll be lucky if she lasts the night' . . . and we're coming in and we're greeting [weeping] and crying and all this carry-on and . . . and they walk in as if . . . 'Come on, Mary, time for your feed' (said very cheerfully), you know, and then they think the mammy and daddy don't know so we'll not tell them, we'll just be cheery all the time and just let things take its course . . . but it's not real, it isn't . . . we would rather be told the truth from beginning to end. We know it's going to be a shock, but all this hiding behind false doors is worse, Philip. (5, p. 40–43)

This account highlighted several aspects of uncertainty that another parent graphically described as 'like being on an emotional roller-coaster'. This was a meaning-laden metaphor that conveyed not only the more obvious sense of emotional peaks and troughs, vulnerability and physical panic, but of being in a situation where control of your life was in the hands of others.

The parents were initially prepared for the possibility, if not the probability, that their child might die as a result of this deterioration in her condition. They tried to prepare themselves and their family for this but found that, while hospital staff were allowed to express a loss of hope for the child's recovery, they were not and were subsequently chastized for 'thinking like that'. It seemed that explicit optimism was expected from parents whatever the severity of their child's condition.

The previously cited mother and father did not appear to be reassured by staff who, perhaps for good reasons, were trying to 'be cheery all the time'. This was not because they wanted everyone to become solemn and dispirited but because this behaviour was undermining what they believed to be their correct understanding of the severity of their child's situation. This led them to question, not their own perceptions of the situation but the motives behind the nurses' actions. They concluded that the nurses were being deliberately dishonest in trying to conceal from them information that they felt that they already knew, and had a right to know.

Uncertainty impeded parents' beginning the process of 'coming to terms' with their child's injuries and future rehabilitation.

> **Father:** I mean, at least if they come up and tell you, you get your shock, you have your wee cry or whatever. . . .
> **Mother:** But you get on with it.
> **Father:** But, you know, you say, 'Right! that's what's happening, carry on,' but this uncertainty . . . (5, p. 43–44)

2.1.5 Concluding comments

Previous studies of parental anxiety and uncertainty have viewed this from a perspective that is essentially psychological and technological. A typical and influential study in this respect is that of Mishel (1983) who saw uncertainty as 'a major perceptual variable' that impeded parents in their 'successful psychological management of the ill child'. Here, I propose an alternative understanding of parents' uncertainty and anxiety that rejects an understanding of these as being context-free, private, subjective possessions. I argue that the parents' experiences of uncertainty and anxiety are best approached, not as aberrations to be 'managed', but as part of the existential dread of being a parent whose child, and thus whose very self, is threatened. Heidegger (1962, p. 329) used the expression 'thrownness' (*Geworfenheit*) to describe how '*Dasein* is something that has been thrown; it has been brought into its "there", but not of its own accord.' Here we gain a sense of what it is to find oneself in a particular existential situation. I believe that the existential question, Why are we here rather than not here? would have been understood by parents who asked 'Why me?', 'Why our child?'. But the answer would surely have eluded them, for there is likely to be none, short of a religious faith, that would have satisfied them. Similarly, I suggest that the idea of 'thrownness' helps to capture the parents' understandings of their child's illness or injury and admission to hospital. This seems particularly helpful where the child's admission was an emergency. One parent described this as she told of how she sat attempting to console another mother in the intensive care unit. This mother's child had been happy and healthy only the previous day, but was now lying very seriously ill in an intensive care unit. The participant mother described how

> I just sat down beside her 'cos there was nothing to say and she turned round to me and said, 'He was sitting up eating jelly and ice-cream yesterday, and now look at him.' (17, p. 75)

Another dimension of a phenomenological understanding of uncertainty and anxiety is that 'thrownness' does not imply a landing, a thrown-on-to-something-firm. Parents described this when they spoke of how the child's illness or injury had left them groundless. They described how 'the bottom had fallen out of their world', how they 'no longer knew where they stood' and how the whole experience had been 'like a dream or nightmare'.

Viewing uncertainty and anxiety as a personal trait or as a particular response to a discrete event also ignores the importance of temporality. This refers to a conception of time where 'temporality is constitutive of being' as opposed to traditional Western notions of 'an endless succession of "nows"' (Leonard, 1989, p. 48–49). This means that a temporal understanding of uncertainty and anxiety takes into account that parents' understandings have been shaped by a past and are projected towards a future. Many parents described how their reflecting back upon the events prior to their child's illness or injury had contributed to their sense of uncertainty and anxiety. They relived the past, asking themselves why; why they hadn't noticed 'something' earlier, why they had left their child 'just for a moment'. 'If only' they had. . . .

The parent's and child's future also helped to constitute parents' present anxiety. This was especially notable in the parents of the children who were likely to have serious future problems, for example children who had been burned or scalded or who had a chronic illness or neurological injury. The nurses in the burns unit were very aware that they seemed to be working within a different time frame from parents. While nurses tended to concentrate upon the present, parents' anxieties and uncertainties were already projected towards the future. As one nurse explained:

> They count years ahead as well. I mean, us, we take it a day at a time, whereas their outlook is x number of years away, and it's difficult to get

them to try and come back and think about what's happening today and tomorrow. (24, p. 13)

A further reason for viewing uncertainty and anxiety ontologically rather than purely cognitively is that parents' embodied, skilled child-care practices are compromised. Parents described the difficulty of carrying out previously unproblematic activities such as feeding or changing their child and I suggest that this was not simply because they lacked sufficient information. Parents had embodied skills and practices that were usually ready-to-hand (Heidegger, 1962) in that they were fluent, unnoticed and transparent, in the way that a cyclist is unaware of his cycling skills while cycling. However, the child's illness or injury and the parent's fears, their anxieties and their new situation made this ready-to-hand mode of involvement break down. In Heidegger's terms, the parent's involvement was now unready-to-hand and the previously familiar was now strange and often threatening. In Chapter 4 the parents' participation in the care of their child is discussed in more detail, but it is appropriate here to describe some of the ways in which parents felt that they were becoming 'like a different parent'.

2.2 ADAPTING TO BECOMING A LIVE-IN PARENT

The parents' accounts suggested that being a live-in parent involved more than simply continuing as before but within the different location of the ward. Parents described their living-in in terms that suggested that this was a period of great change for them. The changes were not only the logistical ones about learning to live in a new environment, but were more fundamentally related to parents' ways of 'being-in-the-world' (Heidegger, 1962). Heidegger uses this expression to indicate that a person's existence (*Dasein*), or being-there, is always a being-in related to world. Benner and Wrubel (1989) further explain that being-in-the-world 'describes how people are involved in situations through their concerns, skills and practical activity' (Benner and Wrubel, 1989, p. 407). A central theme of this book is that living-in involved parents in considerable change and discontinuity that affected the very concerns, skills and practical activities that were so fundamental to their being parents.

2.2.1 Sharing responsibility and care

At home, parents are the child's main source of love, care and nurture. But perhaps of greatest importance for this discussion is that parents have considerable autonomy in relation to the child and therefore they have the right to make decisions affecting almost every aspect of the child's life. Clearly embedded within these ideas of responsibility and rights over the child are the related issues of everyday knowledge of the child, power and the parent's perceived moral adequacy. To highlight parental responsibility is not to suggest, however, that a parent or parents make(s) all of the decisions regarding their child in complete isolation. Parents have background meanings to draw upon and networks of family and friends who may influence their decisions. Similarly, parents may already share the everyday care of the child if the child stays regularly with friends, grandparents or child-minders. It is likely that here however, the sharing is initiated by the parents and remains within their control.

In hospital however, this sharing of the child's care seemed to represent for parents not so much of a sharing as a take-over of responsibility which threatened their sense of autonomy and control over their child and his or her care and treatment. One mother described the above concerns:

> You're not the only one that's responsible when they're in here because there are so many other people that are deciding various things that are going to happen as well, even silly things like when they're going to eat and what they're going to be offered . . . you haven't got the same freedom to do either what you want or what they ask for . . . you have to fit in to what their plans are. (27, Mother 1, p. 9)

This mother's account nicely captured several of the major ways in which parents could feel themselves effectively disempowered and de-skilled. Areas of child care previously the exclusive concern of the parents were now shared, or possibly taken over by 'so many' professionals. This mother also highlighted the concern that even the 'silly things' – everyday and previously unproblematic child care – were now outwith their control.

Normal parenting had previously taken place within the context of the home and family. This gave a particular rhythm and meaning to everyday child-care tasks such as washing, feeding and changing. Parents' domestic lives provided a particular variety and structure to their day, which they reported as being noticeably absent, even within the structure imposed by the rhythms and practices of the hospital itself (Zerubavel, 1979). The loss of this normal routine seemed to rob what nurses viewed as 'homelike' or 'ordinary' tasks of their essential meaning. A mother explained this well when she described how the once simple act of getting her baby's feed ready had been taken over and somehow diminished for her:

> Even putting the kettle on, getting the bottle out of the fridge, that always takes up a few minutes but you're not doing that here. . . . When you say to the nurse, 'Oh, that's him due a feed,' she'll go and get it. . . . It's just not the same. (9, p. 7)

The character of parents' interaction with their child was also affected within the new context of the ward. This was clearly highlighted by mothers who discussed the problem of discipline while their child was in hospital.

2.2.2 Discipline: 'trying to get back to normal'

At the time of the child's admission, discipline was not a pressing issue as any 'bad' behaviour could be attributed to the illness, injury or hospitalization and the child was therefore excused the normal responsibility to behave well. This was evident in this section of a mothers' discussion taken from one of the focus groups:

> **Mother 4:** That's one of the things that frightens me about [my daughter], is her **behaviour**, it's **appalling**.'
> **Mother 2:** But a lot of that's to do with what's wrong with her too. (27, p. 65–66)

This period of grace that the child was allowed was only temporary, however, as parents recognized that their normal disciplinary practices would have to be re-established at some point if they were to be able to 'manage' the child within the ward and subsequently when they returned home. The problem for parents was when and how should this return to normal be done. One mother explained that

> You start wondering about how you're going to manage to discipline them and how do you know when they're well enough to start disciplining them (. . .) and then try to get back to normal. (27, Mother 1, p. 66)

As the child's condition improved, the parents were faced with the problem of how to continue to use their own disciplinary practices. If these were seen as being at variance with the professional ethos of the ward and ward staff, parents were liable to incur staff disapproval at the very least. Paediatric nurse education emphasizes a disciplinary ethic towards children that is based upon calm, reason and explanation. When confronted by children who are being badly behaved, the nurse is encouraged to 'remain unruffled' and of course 'In no circumstances may a nurse hit or smack a child' (Adamson and Hull, 1984, p. 336).

My reason for distinguishing between parents' disciplinary practices and nurses' disciplinary ethos is to bring out what I believe to be an important distinction that helps to make clear the interpretive significance of this discussion of discipline. Parents' disciplinary practices are part of their everyday pattern of child care where their involvement is 'ready-to-hand' (Heidegger, 1962). That is, because of their active involvement with their child and their expertise in the micropractices of discipline, it does not usually show itself as problematic. However, because of parents' altered situation, the normal smooth functioning of their disciplinary practices was compromised. In addition, when these essentially private disciplinary techniques were transposed to a public arena, they came under a more public and moral scrutiny.

The ward was a public arena, with what parents believed to be a pervasive set of moral assumptions, namely a professional ethic of 'correct' child-care practices. Parents were acutely aware that such an ethos was also applicable to them and that they were expected to conform to this. When parents smacked their child in the ward, they believed that their action had incurred the moral disapproval of other parents and the nurses. One mother's experience of what I call the paediatric equivalent of kicking Bambi was widely shared:

> The first time that I smacked her I was **very conscious** of that, but she'd **really** been naughty and she'd got to the stage where she was really testing the limits . . . and the first time that I smacked her hand I felt that everybody had turned round and **aaarrrrgh!** (makes a hands up in horror gesture) . . . you know, 'she smacked a sick child in hospital!' sort of thing. (10, p. 58–59)

Parents also expressed the concern that their disciplinary styles were being constantly scrutinized and judged by nurses. They feared that nurses who disapproved would believe that they did not care properly for their child. One young mother described this:

> You're not wanting to shout at him and threaten him, 'cos you're frightened that they're going to say 'She's not looking after that bairn.' (25, Mother 1, p. 15)

Some parents were also afraid that their disciplining of the child could lead to the child being seen as at risk of being abused and even taken into care. This was highlighted by the case of one mother who was living-in during the period of fieldwork and with whom I had several conversations and an interview. Some nurses told me that they believed her to be 'too rough' in both her disciplining and handling of her toddler son. As this nurse explained:

> **Nurse:** The mum could get a bit rough with Tommy (. . .) she could sort of shake Tommy, throw him down in the cot and things, and that was noticed.
> **PD:** So was there a real fear for his safety?
> **Nurse:** Yes, very much so. (16, p. 44–45.)

These concerns led to the mother being 'seen by' a social worker and subsequently being told to attend a case conference where staff anxieties were expressed. The mother saw this development very much as a strong criticism of her competence and adequacy as a mother and as a veiled threat that her child would not be allowed home as the conditions would not be 'safe', especially in relation to his fragile skin graft site. She was then very aware that her style of parenting was unacceptable within the ward and that staff were assessing her performance to determine whether she had altered her 'behaviour' sufficiently in order to allay their fears concerning the child's eventual discharge. This was one particular illustration of how parents could perceive themselves as being policed by a network of agencies including doctors, nurses, social workers, other parents and even themselves.

The phrase 'seen by' was particularly revealing as parents could presumably be seen by anyone in the ward, in that they were visible. They were also seen by nurses for a variety of reasons. However, this particular sense of 'seen by' carried more disciplinary overtones. Foucault (1973) has described the 'medical gaze' as being significantly different from the gaze of an 'ordinary' observer. This is the gaze of a professional who holds powers to make extremely important decisions and interventions. From this mother's perspective, being 'seen by' the social worker or doctor could have resulted in decisions and interventions being made which would have taken her child from her. I return to the question of nurses' judgements of parents later in this chapter and in Chapter 3. The question of parents living-in under a disciplinary gaze is discussed more fully in Chapter 6.

The previously noted difference in temporal understanding between nurses and parents was also apparent in relation to discipline, with parents expressing more concern for the child's behaviour in the longer term. The parents were concerned that if children were 'ruined' or allowed to 'get away with murder' while in hospital, that this would create serious problems for the family when the child returned home. A mother used this concern to justify her continuing to smack her child within the ward when she felt that this was necessary:

> He gets away with it with the nurses but he's not getting away with it with me, 'cos I've got the wee one back home and if he's going to get away with the likes of pushing other kids about here, and hitting other kids, he's going to think that he's going to get away with it at home. (15, p. 28)

This discussion of discipline shows up how a normal and everyday parental practice was influenced and altered by the social context of the ward. I argue that parents' disciplinary practices are among the most emotive and personal aspects of being a parent. In normal social intercourse, it would be highly inappropriate to suggest, however gently, to friends or other parents that there was something wrong with the ways in which their child was disciplined. Pointing out occasions where they should discipline their child and suggesting how this should be done would be equally unwelcome. Yet within the ward, this was exactly what appeared to occur. Discipline was an issue that revealed wider issues of control and power over the child in hospital and of the importance of the parent's moral identity.

2.2.3 'Learning the ropes'

Although, as I shall show, the nurses had clear ideas of what they expected from live-in parents, this was not openly articulated to the parents themselves. One result of this was that parents were uncertain as to what was expected of them while they were resident, in relation to both their child's care and their own personal comportment.

Parents described mixed experiences of receiving helpful information about living-in. Most parents expressed the view that they were expected to 'pick things up as they went along'. As these parents noted:

> It's all just a case of guesswork, or asking, 'Is it all right if I do this?' . . . to see just what you can and can't do'. (25, Mother 1, p. 6)

> You get told as the days go on what you've done wrong, or what is not hospital policy. (26, Mother 5, p. 14–15)

This was a view shared by many of the nurses who believed that too little explanation was given to parents on admission. One nurse explained that

> I think it's bad that, when parents do come in, I don't think that we lay down to them what we are expecting of them . . . and it's very much, 'There's the locker, the nappies are in there and just get on with it' and I don't always think that they are told exactly what we are expecting from them. (30, Nurse 2, p. 2)

In the absence of any clear guidance regarding what they could or should do while living-in, parents described how the process of 'learning the ropes' became a major task facing the live-in parent during the early part of their stay.

Both my observations and parents' accounts suggested that parents often drew upon the experience and understandings of other parents who were already living-in. They watched them closely to see what they did for their child and took a lead from this example, or asked them directly for information and assistance. There was a greater willingness among parents to approach other parents rather than nurses, as nurses were usually seen as being 'too busy' or 'rushed off their feet' and therefore not to be legitimately interrupted. It may also have been the case that an approach to another parent could have been an opening to try to establish a connectedness or friendship with a fellow resident. A further reason may have been that parents made a positive choice to approach other parents as they believed that they were in fact the best people to guide them as they were undergoing a broadly similar experience.

Commonly, parents described 'learning the ropes' and the rules of living-in as a process of trial and error. They tried to carry on with their normal styles and routines of parenting until such a strategy fell foul of the rules of the ward or hospital policy. The most illustrative example of this trial and error adaptation to living-in on the ward was parents and the ward kitchens. It was clear from listening to parents' accounts of difficulties in this particular area that strong feelings had been aroused. Particularly resented here was the policy in some wards whereby no children or parents were allowed into the ward kitchen. Some wards had a large notice on the kitchen door to this effect but others did not. Parents would often only realize their mistake when 'ticked off' by a nurse who found them in the kitchen trying to get a drink for their child or looking for their baby's feed.

Parents were unhappy about this kind of rule because it put them in the difficult position of ostensibly being in the ward to bring a continuity and normality to the child's stay while being unable to effect this in practice. Parents felt that it was both unrealistic and uncomfortable always to have to request that a nurse go to the kitchen for their every need. In addition to increasing parents' sense of dependence and powerlessness, this practice was seen by parents as casting doubt upon their competence to prepare a feed or pour a drink for their child. The parents who described this problem were also concerned that it placed them in the uncomfortable position of being a nuisance. They now had to make more demands on the nurses' time; time which parents perceived to be very limited. One mother explained this:

> If they're short-staffed, you **really can't** go and ask a nurse to go and make them a bit of toast or get them some juice if they're rushing around doing something else. (27, Mother 1, p. 16)

This requirement to ask nurses to perform simple fetching tasks also made parents feel that nurses might think that the parents themselves were being lazy or unnecessarily demanding. This was clear in the following parent's account:

> You always feel embarrassed to ask someone to do such a thing [make a slice of toast for her child]. . . . It's almost as if you're sitting there saying, Well **I'm** not going to do that, that's **your** job. (27, Mother 1, p. 18)

However, this 'rule' regarding the ward kitchen was not applied rigorously and consistently, which suggested that it served a purpose other than to simply prevent parents from entering the kitchen. I became aware of this when I spoke with one mother whose child had been admitted to a particular ward on numerous previous occasions and who was well known to the staff. She explained that she went into the kitchen as she pleased because she was an 'old hand at this', meaning living-in. She also made the point that she was believed by the nurses to be fully conversant with all of her child's regular treatments and tests and that for this reason the staff trusted in her competence 'just to get on with it'. A mother in a focus group interview expressed a similar view:

> . . . but once you've been in for a while, and . . . certainly I wouldn't have done it the first couple of days . . . but then I got to know that they would allow you (. . .) that you could go and get the juice and you knew how to measure it, we're not stupid . . . you know what you're doing. (27, Mother 4, p. 17)

The issue of access to ward kitchens involved more than simply entry to some 'off-stage' ward area. My interpretation of parents' and nurses' comments on the ward kitchen suggests that these accounts reveal important aspects of wider issues of the development of trust, parental competence and the tension between parents as individuals and the ward as a social collective.

It is possible that this rule was in force not simply to prevent accidents and to preserve the limited stocks of food and drinks, two reasons given by nurses. The rule also recognized some parents as having reached a standard of competence acceptable to nurses and thus to be trusted in this area. Analogies may be drawn here between this gradual allowing of access to the kitchen to certain parents and the system of allocating prisoners the status of 'trusty'. The question of access to the kitchen also highlighted the difficulties that nurses faced in reconciling the needs of individual parents with what they saw as the wider issues of the smooth running of the ward and of trying to ensure equity of treatment.

This latter point was brought out in one nurse's account of how she had displeased a parent by not allowing her to go to the kitchen to make her child a slice of toast for his supper. Although from the mother's perspective this was clearly a reasonable request unreasonably denied, the nurse argued that because the staff were very busy and did not have time to make toast for any of the other children who might have wanted it, her refusal was therefore justified. As the nurse explained:

> I said, (. . .) 'Not all mums are here to make toast for all the kids and we don't have time to make it for them all.' . . . I said it in a nice way. (25, tape counter 382)

2.2.4 Concluding comments

I have shown that parents' early days in the ward were characterized and shaped by uncertainty, confusion and attempts to adapt to being a parent of a hospitalized child in this new situation. Not only were parents largely unaware of how they were expected to function as live-in parents but they also believed themselves to have been divested of some of the responsibility for their child that they believed to be an essential part of being a parent. Parents' accounts also suggested that tensions between them and the nurses could quickly arise.

A previously stated phenomenological assumption that underpins this study is that meaning is co-created. As Allen *et al.* explain: 'Meaning resides neither solely within the individual nor solely within the situation. Meaning is a transaction between the two so that the individual both constitutes and is constituted by the situation' (Allen *et al.* 1986, p. 28).

In order to understand more fully the relational nature of parents' early experiences, it was important to examine also the nurses' understandings. As I stress in Chapter 7, this was not done in order to perform 'ironies' by using one set of accounts to prove or disprove the 'truth' of the other (Silverman, 1985, p. 20–21). I now explore the nurses' perceptions and expectations of live-in parents, focusing particularly on how nurses initially viewed parents and how family and parental identity came to be socially created within the context of the hospital and ward.

2.3 NURSES' PERCEPTIONS OF LIVE-IN PARENTS

I elicited nurses' perceptions of parents who lived-in and their understandings of paediatric nursing practices in relation to these parents. We discussed parents in general and individual parents with whom they were working at present or with whom they had worked in the past. Typically, the nurses told stories that emphasized the individuality of parents. They prefaced many of their responses to questions by saying that their opinion or approach in a given situation 'depended on the parents'. They claimed that it was neither possible nor desirable to 'lump them all together' into a homogenous group.

In their accounts of working with live-in parents and of the relationship that developed between themselves and the parents, it emerged clearly that nurses regarded the individual parent as being a critical determinant. This was most commonly expressed when nurses spoke of the importance that they attributed to what they referred to as the parent's 'personality'. Two nurses explained this:

> Obviously there are personalities involved [in the development of nurse–parent relationships]. I mean, if you don't like the person, I mean, if you don't like them and *vice versa* (. . .) it's going to be . . . . . . and do you say, 'I'm not going near that child 'cos the mother's there; I'm going to hold off as long as possible?'

> It's the personality of the parent. When you get situations like that [where there are tensions between the parents and ward staff] it tends to be definitely the personality of the person.

Although themes of parents' individuality and personalities occurred frequently in nurses' accounts, they also described other factors that shaped their understandings of and interactions with live-in parents. Some of these factors developed during the parents' stay in the ward, for example nurses' judgements of how 'well' parents participated in their child's care. Other influential factors were more immediate.

2.3.1 Nurses' expectations: co-operation, competence and character

Parents' child-care practices were important in shaping nurses' views. So too, were aspects of parents' personal lives, especially where these became highly visible within the ward, for example, where a young single mother had 'boyfriends' visiting her. I explore this question of parents' moral identities in greater detail in Chapter 3.

Nurses' perceptions were influenced by the expectations that they held concerning live-in parents. Nurses described these expectations when they discussed parent participation, how they assessed parents and what they found to be advantageous and disadvantageous in the presence of live-in parents. Interpretation of these sections of the nurses' accounts revealed recurrent themes that emphasized the importance for nurses of parental co-operativeness, competence and character. While these were not always viewed as being static and unchangeable qualities, they were seen as being important determinants of the 'success' of a parent's stay in hospital.

The nurses described their expectation of parental co-operativeness in general terms and also through their detailing of the kinds of tasks that they expected parents to undertake while living-in. This was also alluded to in nurses' more direct criticisms of parents who they felt were 'abusing' the hospital by living-in and not 'pulling their weight'.

Nurses expected parents to co-operate with them as it was felt that one of the main reasons why parents chose to stay in hospital with their child was to 'help them get better'. From the nurses' perspective, the clear way to achieve this was for parents to work in harmony and co-operation with them and with their plans for the child's care. This co-operativeness was best expressed by parents who showed a willingness to 'help out'. Helping out had both positive and negative dimensions. Positively helping out involved the parents actually carrying out some of the child's daily care. Typically this was what I call 'basic mothering' activities, for example, washing, feeding, changing, occupying and amusing the child. However, as the child's length of stay in hospital increased or if it was thought that the parents would be involved in more long-term care of the child at home, this helping out would be expected to include tasks which might initially have been considered to be 'too technical' or exclusively nurses' work, for example nasogastric feeding.

The nurses felt strongly that a willingness to help with the child's 'basic care' was expected and that the absence of such willingness could signify a problem at least, or perhaps even some form of psychosocial disturbance on the part of the mother or mother and child. As these nurses suggested:

Well, any **ordinary** parent, you would expect them to do their own child's care. (8, p. 3)

We seem to expect that they will, if they're going to stay, help with the care (. . .) that they're not just going to sit there and be bystanders and if a person for some reason doesn't want to participate, if they want to be in all day but don't want to participate, it can seem to make a blockage. . . .' (7, p. 32) [I think that when this nurse says 'make a blockage', she means 'create problems'.]

Nurses also expected that live-in parents would organize their routine of living-in in such a way as to enable them to become a better source of help both to their child and to the nurses. This involved the parents 'fitting-in' with the ward routine in such a way as to be there at the times when the nurses felt that they would be most needed. Commonly this was in the morning when their child was getting up, at mealtimes and at night when the child was going to bed. There were obvious advantages for the nurses in having parents help at these times since they were typically 'basic mothering' periods.

It would be a mistake, however to conclude from this that nurses were cynically 'using' parents to carry out unpopular, unexciting, basic care while they undertook more preferred, exciting, technical tasks. The nurses, as well as most parents, professed that it was parents themselves who 'knew the child best'. Therefore, at mealtimes for example, a parent was usually more likely to be able to encourage a child to eat and drink than a nurse. Similarly, nurses were aware that younger children, especially, can become very upset if they awoke in strange surroundings without a familiar parent present (Lovell-Davis, 1986; Thornes, 1987). As one nurse observed:

> Obviously they don't want to leave the child alone any time they are awake. (. . .) Some of the parents are called at night 'cos the child gets very agitated (. . .) 'cos they are so attached to their parents . . . they get so upset at night if their parents are not there. (21, p. 2)

A tension that seemed to arise here was that while the nurses claimed to value parents' expertise and particular knowledge regarding their child, this was not always visible in the nurses' practices in ways which assured parents that their knowledge was being truly valued. This may help to account for the finding that many parents described their role within the ward as being to 'help out' the busy nurses.

Parents who the nurses felt did not 'help out' adequately or appropriately were criticized for being lazy, devious or for having 'fun' by abusing the 'privilege' of living-in and 'treating the place like a hotel' or 'like Butlin's Holiday Camp'. The nurses distinguished between these parents and others whom they judged to be overawed by the strangeness of the ward and by the traumatic nature of their child's illness or injury. One nurse described how she 'sussed out' parents who she felt were not co-operating and caring in the way that she believed that live-in parents should:

> **Nurse:** You can suss them out almost immediately, the ones that aren't there all day but are caring and the ones that aren't there all day 'cos they can't be bothered, I can think of an example of that, too. . . .
> **PD:** What would the differences be in what they would do?
> **Nurse:** Leave it to the nurses. Not . . . – OK, we're paid for the job anyway but . . . you know – right, well . . . they'd come in not at mealtimes, they time it: 'Oh, what's that, half-twelve? Right, I'll go along now for a wee while . . . when the dinners are over'. (16, p. 54–55)

This perception that parents were expected to be there because they had specific work to do suggested a particular understanding on the part of some nurses regarding their relationship with live-in parents. It seemed that for these nurses, parents were essentially part of the workforce. Through a concentration upon the 'basic mothering' elements of the child's care, the parent's place in the workforce seemed to be near the bottom of any occupational hierarchy. This expectation of parents as workers was stressed by another nurse who described how parents could be deemed to be unco-operative by not being there when they were needed:

> You do get the odd parent living-in who's not at all interested, is never in the ward when you need them, whatever you've done, taken the child away

to take blood, I mean if Mum's there she's there to comfort the kid afterwards, and it's the jobs that Mum's going to do better than us 'cos they've
got the time to sit there. (11, p. 10)

The nurses did not expect parents to possess a level of technical competence
regarding nursing or medical procedures. However, they did expect that 'intelligent' parents, as they described them, would be able to understand information
about their child that was given to them and that they could learn particular skills
in the future if it were thought that this was necessary. The 'intelligence' of
parents was often referred to by the nurses, as they described how they would
assess parents in relation to how they might participate in their child's care while
in hospital. This is shown in these sections of accounts:

> A lot of it comes down to your initial assessment of . . . . . . yes, how capa-
> ble you think that they are of being able to handle that . . . uhuh (. . .) I'm
> kind of coming on to . . . I don't like to say it, but intelligence in a way . . .
> you assess, like, sometimes you're speaking to parents and they're really not
> taking in what you're saying, not so much because it's tragic information
> that you're giving them, but because of their understanding . . . they don't
> have the capacity. . . . 30, Nurse 2, p. 6–7)

> **Nurse:** When you explain . . . dare I say the parent's level of intelligence?'
> **PD:** You can dare say anything that you like.
> **Nurse:** Some of them are a bit more . . . slower than . . . you know, you try
> to explain to them what the child needs and what is going to be happening
> and things like that and they don't really grasp it . . . don't seem to under-
> stand. (21, p. 20)

It became clear that the nurses were uncomfortable, almost apologetic, in discussing their thoughts regarding what they described as the parents' 'intelligence'.
I also gained the impression that they felt that I would disapprove of their
comments. This could have been because I was known to the nurses as both
a researcher and a nurse teacher and was thus identified with a system which
had labelled such assessments illegitimate. I can best explain this comment
by briefly examining the ways in which nursing and, in a curiously relevant
way, flight attendants, have conceptualized 'good' and 'bad' patients and
passengers, for this relates directly to the legitimacy of nurses' judgements of
parents.

Hochschild's (1983) study of flight attendants' management of emotions
described how the attendants had a different vocabulary to describe 'bad' passengers. While they would describe 'bad' passengers as being 'obnoxious', 'out-
rageous' or 'irates', their supervisors spoke instead of an 'uncontrolled' passenger
(Hochschild, 1983, p. 110–111). I suggest that there is a similar approach in
nursing to what might be called 'problem' patients or parents. While nurses may
speak privately of some parents using a more derogatory range of epithets, the

'official' or 'professional' view represented by senior nurses, managers and educators is that such patients are merely 'unpopular' or 'non-compliant recipients of health care' (Armitage, 1980). Hochschild (1983) argued that the flight attendant's right to be angry with or to criticize a passenger was linguistically 'smuggled out of the discourse' (Hochschild, 1983, p. 112) through the use of euphemism. This helps to explain why nurses may have felt that any critical or negative judgements of parents required to be expressed very carefully.

It was widely expected that parents would immediately be able to carry out the normal 'basic mothering' tasks that they would usually carry out at home, provided that the child's condition was not so serious as to have transformed these once normal tasks into more technical procedures. It was also expected that parents would understand information given to them by the nurses and that they would act 'appropriately' on the basis of such information. When parents did not accept nurses' advice in this way, their competence and desire to do what was best for their child was called into question.

An illustration of this was the recurrent theme in the nurses' accounts of the parents who flouted their advice or who asked the 'stupidest questions' related to their child's care. One nurse gave a typical example of this kind of story:

> It's like certain children with cleft palate and soft diet and why it's involved and some parents, you explain it once or twice and they say, 'Can the child have crisps [potato chips]?' . . . and it does get to you . . . things like that and you think, am I explaining myself right, 'cos I have done it so many times before and everybody else understood and why are **these** parents not taking it in?'. (21, p. 20–21)

Some nurses would ascribe such unwillingness or inability to understand and co-operate competently to the parent's level of 'intelligence', claiming that they were simply unable to understand what was being expected of them. This was similar to Strong's (1979a) finding that doctors in paediatric clinics tended to 'sum up' mothers as being 'bright' or 'dim', 'intelligent' or 'unintelligent', 'sensible' or 'worriers' as part of a wider evaluation of their moral character (Strong, 1979a, p. 156).

A second explanation which nurses offered was that the parents might have experienced such trauma and anxiety that they were temporarily unable to understand and respond appropriately. However, I suggest that this 'justification' was only acceptable initially. After the event, parents were expected to have 'come to terms' with the situation and to be once more receptive and responsive to the nurses' suggestions regarding their co-operation. A third explanation of parents' apparent lack of understanding, which will be discussed more fully in relation to parents' moral adequacy and identity, was that the nurses may have believed that a particular parent 'didn't really care' about their child and therefore had no real interest in understanding aspects of the child's care.

Interestingly, few of the nurses who were interviewed described ways in which nurses' communicative approaches with parents could have been partly responsible for the reported failures in parental understanding. The previously cited extract (21, p. 20–21) may seem to be an example of a nurse's reflection upon her success in communication but I would argue that this should be interpreted more as a self-justificatory 'I've made it clear to everyone else that I've explained it to, so it's your [the parent's] fault for not understanding this time'. Several nurses felt that parents were not adequately involved in discussions as to what their role in hospital should be. One group of nurses made this point emphatically during a focus group interview:

> **PD:** So . . . do you make clear to parents who are coming in what they are there for?
> **All five nurses in group (emphatically):** No . . . No! (29, p. 4)

This description of nurses' expectations and understandings of live-in parents has suggested ways in which nurses' expectations influenced parents' early days in the ward and their transition to becoming live-in parents. However, as I have previously argued, becoming a live-in parent was not merely a matter of carrying on with normal parenting activities within a different setting. Other important questions of self and identity were involved.

One of the important tasks facing live-in parents during the initial period was the establishment of their moral and social identity within the ward. In the following section I show that for nurses, parents' identities within the ward were revealed more obliquely than directly. Exceptions to this were where, for example, visitation rights to a child were openly complicated by the separation, divorce or explicit ill-feeling between parents (Coucouvanis and Solomons, 1983). In these cases, the issue of who was a legitimate parent was more manifest than latent.

In the following section, the intention is to reveal the everyday meanings of being a 'parent' and 'family' as problematic. This is done by questioning the concepts in a way which helps to illustrate how they came to be created within the context of the ward.

2.3.2 Creating parents and family

Much of the previously cited literature on parent participation and family-centred care assumes that the concepts of 'parent' and 'family' are unproblematic, in that parents and family are easily identified through their obvious kinship with the child. This situation may have arisen because the concepts of 'parent' and 'family' are more commonly defined and extolled than examined as to their use and meaning, particularly within paediatric nursing. If the only question asked is 'Who are parents and family?' it is likely that mere definitions of kinship or lists of traits will result. Here, I follow what I suggest are more fruitful ways of looking at parents and families.

In this discussion, I draw upon the work of Gubrium and Buckholdt (1982a) and Gubrium and Lynott (1985) to help illuminate the more problematic dimensions of the concepts of 'family' and 'parent'. I also show that this issue has important implications for how nurses view live-in parents and consequently how they help to create the conditions of their stay in hospital. Rather than attempting to describe family by defining who is or is not family according to predefined criteria that usually involve kinship, Gubrium and Lynott (1985) suggest that it may be more useful to consider the family assignment process itself as being the definition. As they note: 'Family therefore becomes how and to what family is assigned, focusing our attention in its signs and signification' (Gubrium and Lynott, 1985, p. 133).

I describe how nurses' ideas regarding parents and family were constituted through their understandings of both social relationships and parents' perceived moral adequacy. I then examine the influence that nurses' interpretations of these concepts have for the initiation and subsequent development of nurse–parent–family relationships. I did not ask the nurses specific questions regarding how they viewed the concept of family or whom they considered to be family or non-family. However, there were sections in the nurses' accounts where their discussions of increasing parental presence and involvement, and their descriptions of their interactions with particular parents, were interpreted as revealing their understandings of this issue.

(a) Marginalized family: being 'out of it'

It was noteworthy that very few of the nurses interviewed mentioned fathers as parents. This undoubtedly reflected the fact that it was mostly mothers who lived-in with their child (cf. Knafl and Dixon, 1984). Where a father did try to live-in with the mother, he often suggested that he was relatively ignored by nurses. One young father who was living-in with his girlfriend, the child's mother, described this sense of feeling excluded:

> I don't think they like the fathers staying in with the bairns, 'cos they'll not do nothing to find them a room. (25, p. 101)

A nurse echoed this sentiment as she described how she saw a parent's 'typical day':

> A lot seem to end up just sitting there and reading their own books and magazines . . . a lot of mums actually sit and do their knitting, and dads, actually I feel that dads are more out of it even still. (7, p. 10)

The point made here by this father was an interesting illustration of how the hospital as an organization helped to shape the concept of 'parent' in such a way that this became virtually synonymous with 'mother'. The father was referring to the difficulty that he faced in getting accommodation within the hospital's admittedly limited residential facilities for parents. This facility was called the 'Mothers' Unit', which by its very title seemed to exclude the possibility of there being live-in fathers.

The strangeness of this idea of fathers being equal parents with mothers was reiterated in the information leaflet describing the Mothers' Unit. This stated that 'in exceptional circumstances two parents may stay'. Another feature of the organization of the hospital that helped to create the concept of mother alone as parent were the other facilities which were afforded to mothers but which were denied to other family members. For example, a live-in mother could be given a meal pass which gave her access to the Staff Cafeteria, the only place in the hospital where a choice of meals was available. The Mothers' Unit information leaflet again stressed that 'the meal pass can only be used by the person to whom it has been issued. Unfortunately we are unable to cater for families in this cafeteria.' Although this was the rule regarding meal passes for live-in parents it was observed that where a father was staying-in with his child for long periods, some nurses would try to obtain a meal pass for him also. However, this had to be done surreptitiously and with the understanding that this was an arrangement that should not be widely broadcast.

It would be simplistic and unhelpful here to attribute motives of malice or lack of caring to the hospital, for the simple logistics of accommodating and catering for families within the confines of a very old and relatively small building were very real. However, the effect of these organizational policies seemed to be to set boundaries for the 'socially discretionary' (Gubrium and Lynott, 1985) relegation of fathers and other members of families to a marginal role.

When fathers were seen as being parents in a different sense from mothers, this could reflect traditional societal concepts of maternal and paternal roles. For example, mothers were expected to carry out the 'basic mothering' types of care, while fathers were given the opportunity to undertake activities more in keeping with their assumed paternal place. One mother described the hurt that she felt when the 'special occasion' of her badly scalded son being able to get out of bed for the first time for a cuddle was saved for her husband to enjoy:

> He said, 'My dad gave me a cuddle today!' . . . 'cos it was the first time he was out the bed and **I was jealous** . . . and I was hurt 'cos it wasn't me . . . and then at the weekend there the nurse says, 'Is daddy coming in today?' and I says, 'Not till later on,' and she says, 'Well, when daddy comes in we'll get him to sit on the chair and give daddy a big cuddle,' . . . and I thought, why not me?. . . Supposing I couldn't lift him out, I mean, they could have done it and I could have sat there with the bairn . . . but . . . 'We'll get daddy when he comes in' . . . and that really hurt me, because I feel he's more my bairn than he is Robert's, you know, he's **my bairn.** . . . (25, Mrs A, p. 86–87)

If, as I suggest, fathers were not assigned as parents by nurses in the same way that mothers were, they were not the only family members in this situation. To illustrate this, it is useful to compare the competing perspectives of parents and nurses regarding how family was constituted. The following account is worth citing at length as it is illustrative of how the social forms of parent and family were created within the ward. Here, a young mother described an occasion that had angered and upset her:

> She [one of the nurses] has treated me like a bairn from when I came in here ... and I mean, if it wasn't for my mum and my auntie – when Ben was first brought in he was tied down the whole time (. . .) and my mum and my auntie and my gran and her pal had come through to see the bairn a few days after it happened . . . and he was lying and his feet and his hands were blue and my mum went away to call for a nurse to come in and check him, and they were smacking him . . . they smacked his bare bum, they shook him about and he **still** wouldn't wake up . . . and they finally went . . . they had to go and get another nurse to come and help get him awake (. . .) I had to sit with him all night to keep him awake . . . and my mum came in the next day and Nurse Crimson said, 'Look, you can't go in that cubicle.' My mum says, 'Why not?' 'Infections. You've been on public transport. It's only the parents.' Mum turned round and says, 'I'm on public transport but his dad's on public transport when he comes through [visits], buses, trains and taxis the same as me . . . his clothes are getting infected outside and he's still getting in,' . . . and she says, 'Well, it's parents only.' And she come in and said, 'I've just been explaining to your mother that she can't come in.' I says, 'What for?' She says, 'Because she's been on public transport, and it's for the sake of infections,' and I said, 'Well, my man's [husband's] doing exactly the same thing.' . . . I says, 'Look, I don't care what you think, if it wasn't for my mum and my auntie, that bairn would be dead, because nobody was paying attention to him!' (. . .) I says, 'Do you think I'm going to sit in here and let my mum sit out there and try and talk through the door . . . when I could have my mum in here beside her grandson?' . . . . . . 'OK then,' . . . she says, 'Right, fair enough,' and my mum came in, and she washed her hands . . . with the soap, then with the Hibiscrub, then soap, then Hibiscrub . . . and she done that every time she came in just in case. (. . .) She came in, she put her gown on, and she hardly went near him (. . .) and ever since then it's been sort of . . . nark, nark, nark, every time she [Nurse Crimson] sees me. (15, p. 34–38)

This account highlighted several of the factors which nurses believed to be important and which thus became constitutive of parent and family identity within the ward. Of pivotal importance here was Gubrium and Buckholdt's argument that 'Who the "real" family is to everyone concerned is not just a matter of semantics. It meaningfully organizes the ongoing practices of staff's and patients' relating to relatives and acquaintances' (Gubrium and Buckholdt, 1982a, p. 82).

From the outset this mother did not feel that she was being accorded the respect and status of parent by the nurses. She was being 'treated like a bairn' because of her age and demeanour. I suggest here that this mother felt strongly that her mother, auntie, gran and even her 'pal' were 'real' family, not solely on the basis of kinship but because of their actions and expressed concern for Ben. They were the ones who had 'paid attention to him' and intervened to protect Ben when he had seemed to turn blue, thus in his mother's eyes, 'saving his life'. When the nurse tried to prohibit the grandmother from entering the child's cubicle the following day this revealed a discrepancy and tension between professional and parental perceptions of 'family'.

The nurse tried to constitute family on a narrowly defined kinship basis by suggesting that it was only parents who were allowed into the cubicle, thus excluding the grandmother from this privileged role that would have allowed her access. Ironically for the mother, the child's father would have been considered to be a more legitimate 'parent' and allowed in, despite the fact that from the mother's perspective he would have been of no help to her at all. Indeed on one night in the ward he had visited and begun to hit her. Staff were forced to call the police to remove him. This suggests that for parents, the question of family was not so much one of kinship as of the help and support received from those who might occupy this position. I return to other aspects of this issue in Chapter 5's discussion of parents' contact with family and friends.

The nurse's response to the mother and grandmother's claim to sufficient 'familyness' was to suggest that by staking this claim Gran was potentially endangering the child. This is a powerful injunction to counter, for as Smith (1989, p. 149) has observed from his own experiences as a parent of a hospital-ized child: 'To attempt to dismiss the medical view of one's own child exposes us to charges of gross neglect and almost criminal irresponsibility'. The nurse tried to subvert the mother's idea of family by her suggestion that anyone but the biological parents could somehow be a source of infection. However such a claim and the rationale offered in its support seemed so clearly absurd to the mother and grandmother that they had no hesitation in defying the order. Although Gran could not make herself the child's parent, she tried to nullify the nurse's criteria for her exclusion by adopting the cubicle hygiene practices of the nurses and parents who were allowed admission.

It would be easy to gloss linguistically and professionally over this mother's narrative by labelling her a 'non-compliant recipient of health care' (Armitage, 1980). However, as I reflect back upon our interview and consider her way of being as a parent and how this was perceived by staff and others, I feel that she was not simply being difficult. She was literally being herself, as she had been defined by staff and others.

(b) Who are 'family' in family-centred care?

A central tenet of the move towards 'family-centred care' has been that paedi-atric nurses must view as the focus of their care, not solely the child but the child's family, friends and relations (Shelton *et al.*, 1987). Indeed the term family-centred care can often appear so all-encompassing that no one is excluded from its remit. This is not an issue of purely academic interest. Gubrium and

Buckholdt stress that 'the familism question is far from merely definitional. Definitions soon run up against events and activities where resolution of the question is practical, an ongoing, concrete but meaningful issue of relating to families' (Gubrium and Buckholdt, 1982a, p. 86).

One example of the difficulty faced by nurses was that they had to create some system of priority for working with families. At a purely practical and logistic level, treating all family and friends as being equally welcome could create difficulties. As one nurse observed:

> Actually physically getting in and doing what you need to be doing, it can really sometimes be quite awkward. It may not be too bad if there's just parents, but if there are other relatives involved, you know, if you've got four or five round the bed you can't seem to find your patient among them, and you're getting a wee bit . . . you do get tired of having them all there and having to say excuse me to get past, excuse me till I get the charts, excuse me till I get . . . you know, it grates. (7, p. 42–43)

Another nurse, in her discussion of dealing with parents and relatives illustrated this point when she spoke of the perceived disadvantages that could accompany what she called 'complete, open visiting':

Nurse: Chaos, absolute chaos at mealtimes.
PD: Is that just the volume of people, or are there other things?'
Nurse: Weekends are **hell**, you know. . . . You're admitting, maybe a traumatic injury at the weekend, the place is stowed [crowded] out with people. . . . You go up to do the meals and the playroom, you'd think a bomb had hit it. . . . Don't get me wrong, the playroom is to be played in . . . but a lot of the time, it's in-patients who should use it, not all these off the streets who come. . . . One evening I went up, we were short-staffed, we had a lot to do, and I think three adults and five children arrived to see a child on bed rest. Well, they just descended on to the playroom . . . one adult was visiting the child . . . and I said, 'Are you all visiting?' . . . 'Uhuh.' . . . So I said, 'Would you please leave the playroom?' And within 10 minutes they'd all gone home (laughs). I mean, some of the time you have to . . . I mean, I said to the auxiliary, I said, 'We're not here to tidy up after them', but you just get so worn out with continual demands by people coming off the street. (19, p. 9–11)

Such accounts showed clearly the dangers of assuming that phrases such as 'family-centred care' are unproblematic for nurses both in their fundamental philosophy and in their practical implications. The first nurse's account speaks of 'her patient' as being distanced and hidden from her by parents and relatives. There is no sense that this family group is her point of caring contact. They are rather, a physical and possibly metaphorical impediment between her and the legitimate object of her nursing practices, the child.

The second nurse's account suggests a difficulty for the nurse in focusing her attentions on the immediate needs of the child and his kinship parents while also being expected to 'spread' this attention over a wider circle of family and friends. It seemed from this account that the wider circle of family and friends had been perceived largely in terms of their nuisance value. They physically took up space and make the ward or bedside areas look crowded or 'stowed out', they disrupted the orderliness of the ward, for example at mealtimes, and they created untidiness which nurses or other staff had to tidy up. There was also an element in this nurse's account that suggested that extended family and friends were not seen as having the same legitimacy as 'immediate family'. They were not seen as being truly within this nurse's construction of 'family'. They were, in a vivid image of disengagement and unrelatedness, merely people who had 'come off the street'.

For this nurse, the presence of extended family was an indication, not of family cohesiveness and closeness at a time of great stress, but of family chaos and general disorganization. This was particularly clearly demonstrated when the nurse described her perceptions of one family, 'the Joneses', where the parents were both sharing the living-in as the father was unemployed. The grandfather had also decided to stay in the corridor outside the intensive care unit when the child had first been admitted. As there was no accommodation available, he slept in his car at night. The nurse described this situation as she saw it:

> They're all different, and. . . . The Smiths from last weekend, for instance, that mum and dad were just so sorry, they just couldn't believe that it had happened to them. . . . I think you have a different rapport all together with them from . . . what can I say, from the households that you know are so rough-and-tumble, you know, because you do get the mothers who care, who can't believe that it's happened to them, whereas you get the . . . I'm sorry but the Joneses, who . . . are just harum-scarum, just racing around . . . the young people . . . the mother, father, **even the grandfather**, they were just racing everywhere, you know they are away in the car and they're all in the car and they're sleeping in, the kids are sleeping in the car, and you know that their . . . turmoiled life . . . (19, p. 15–16)

2.3.3 Concluding comments

This section has suggested that concepts such as 'parent' and 'family' are more problematic than has previously been acknowledged in the literature regarding parent participation or family-centred care. I have tried to show how nurses understood 'parent' and 'family' both socially and morally. I argue that this has important implications for the practice of paediatric nursing, particularly for the grounding and development of relationships between live-in parents, families and nurses. Organizational influences and nurses' practices were highlighted that perpetuated the idea that caring for children and sick members of the family was the almost exclusive preserve and responsibility of mothers.

I have developed, particularly in relation to nurses, Gubrium and Buckholdt's (1982a) suggestion that it might be more illuminating to examine how 'family' is assigned. To show this I discussed how nurses and parents understood the terms 'family' and 'parent', rather than try to arrive at a single kin- or trait-based definition.

The nurses used both social and moral criteria in assigning who was or was not, a proper parent, immediate family, or a significant other. Nurses seemed to value the more traditional forms of family where parents were husband and wife and where parents' relationships were stable. It seemed particularly important that parents' relationships were free from any complications that could adversely impinge upon or complicate the smooth running of the ward, the nurses' work or relationships with the family.

2.4 SUMMARY

In this chapter I have explored the experience of becoming a live-in parent, uncovering situational, ontological and social dimensions of this process. Although parents often gave particular reasons for wanting to live-in with their child, the strong impression given was that this was not a real choice or decision. The need to be with their child at this time is more primordial than can be understood through the language of rational decision-making.

Parents' entry into this situation was often traumatic. Many of the children had developed acute illnesses or sustained serious injuries and had been admitted as emergencies. The 'thrownness' that parents experienced meant anxiety, confusion, uncertainty, fear, disorientation and a threat to their very being as parents. This threat was present in the guilt and self-reproach which parents experienced and in the fear that their child, and thus the parent within themselves, might actually die.

Parents had to adjust, not only to a physical environment that was strange and often frightening, but to a situation where their ready-to-hand mode of involvement with their child was compromised. Their involvement now had to take into account the influence of others, particularly doctors and nurses. Parents also found that many of their everyday child-care practices had suddenly become unfamiliar and problematic.

I suggest that parents' accounts of their admission and initial period of living-in offer a valuable insight into the ways in which their being-in-the-world as parents changed. Recall how parents described the unreality of this situation, how they felt that no parent other than one who had experienced this could understand, and how they felt that they would never be the same again as a result of this experience.

It is important to recognize however, that becoming a live-in parent was not a purely private and personal transition. Parents became live-in parents in a situation where their meanings and practices were influenced and indeed co-created by others. I have shown that nurses played a significant part in shaping parents' understandings of themselves as live-in parents.

I have introduced the question of parents' moral identity and of the 'good parent'. Parents described how they tried to be a good parent within the context of the ward and nurses similarly explained how they used social and moral criteria to create proper parents and family. This was an important issue and a more detailed exploration offers a clearer understanding of parents' lived experience and of the nature of their relationship with nurses.

Kierkegaard (1956, p. 217–218) suggested that 'pausing is not sluggish repose. Pausing is also movement.' Before moving forward, I want to pause, to re-focus on the parents and to dwell with the story of one mother who kept a brief diary during her stay which she shared with me. In it she wrote:

Only now, after six days in the hospital, am I beginning to feel at ease. It's like living in a goldfish bowl. After the accident my confidence is shattered and simple tasks like changing nappies, feeding and giving drinks are a nightmare, at first I felt as if I was continually being watched by nursing staff. (. . .) I feel so helpless not being able to help him get better and only my love and company to give. (. . .) I feel totally devastated about the accident and know I'm surviving on coffee and nerves. The Mothers' Unit is adequate but the thought of going up to bed at night and usually finding a different mother in the next bed is off-putting. It's a pity it wasn't single rooms, somewhere you could retreat to, even if only to wind down. Don't get me wrong, I don't know how I would even begin to cope if I couldn't stay here, knowing even at night, a phone call from the ward and within two minutes I can be beside him, settling him.

ACKNOWLEDGEMENT

This chapter first appeared as Darbyshire, P. (1994) Parenting in public: parental participation and involvement in the care of their hospitalized child, in *Interpretive Phenomenology as Theory and Method*, (ed P. Benner), Sage Publications, Inc., Newbury Park, CA, p. 185–210 (© by Sage Publications, Inc.). Reprinted by permission of Sage Publications, Inc.

The moral imperative: being a 'good parent' | 3

3.1 INTRODUCTION

In this chapter I discuss the major theme of being a good parent. Clearly this concept does not imply that parents were not 'good' prior to living-in. Rather it suggests that the live-in parent was under pressure to establish their moral adequacy and identity within the context of the ward.

I show that the parents felt strongly that they were expected to be good parents in several senses. Nurses expected them to be good in the more instrumental sense of being competent, useful and helpful to ward staff. Parents could show this in the ways in which they assisted in the care of their child. They were also expected to be good in their more personal ways of being, in their motives, both announced and assumed, in their demeanour, in their character and in what nurses repeatedly referred to as their 'personality'.

Parents' accounts suggested that they held an idealized image of the good mother which influenced their understanding of how they should think and behave while in hospital. This ideal may have been influenced by wider societal images of parenthood (Ruddick, 1989; Richardson, 1991) and also, more specifically, through the context of the ward itself. This image, and the difficulties which parents faced as they tried to attain this arguably unattainable 'ideal state' leads to an exploration of the anxiety and guilt which parents often expressed as they strove to become the good mothers that were expected.

From the interpretation of the parents' accounts I describe a range of strategies through which parents sought to establish their moral identity and worth as 'good parents' in relation to both their character and competence. Moving then to focus on the nurses' accounts, I describe how parents' moral identities within the ward were shaped by nurses' perceptions and approaches. I also show, however, that the shaping of parents' moral identities was not the rather static event of 'labelling' which previous studies have suggested (see Kelly and May, 1982).

3.1.1 Establishing a moral purpose

No parents suggested that they had been put under any explicit or subtle 'moral pressure' to live-in with their child, for example by a nurse suggesting that this was the only course of action which a 'good' parent would choose. This contrasts with Carpenter's (1980) study where two parents complained of such 'emotional blackmail'. Typically, live-in parents came to the ward with only vague ideas that they were there to help their child and the ward staff. Parents had only a diffuse idea regarding the imagined qualities and attributes that a good parent should possess and demonstrate. As two mothers in a group interview noted:

> **Mother 1:** . . . because everybody wants to be the ideal mother like they are in the adverts (laughs).
> **Second mother:** Yeah, coping with the crises and remaining calm and cool. (27, p. 67)

Parents also described several more specific moral dimensions of the initial part of their stay in the ward. It seemed important for parents to establish that they had a clear purpose for wishing to live-in with their child and also to give visible signals that they cared about their child. This was not for themselves, but more for the benefit of others, most importantly the nurses and other parents in the ward. This purpose usually involved the parents' expressed desire to be with their child and to be helpful, thus showing their 'goodness'. As one parent colloquially noted, she wanted the nurses to know that she was there to be of functional value and to appreciate that she was:

> . . . a good mum to Alan, that I'm not just in here for a heat out of the cold, right, do you follow that? (6, p. 28)

There was an impression, given not only by nurses but by other parents, that there was a definite morally acceptable way for parents to behave when they elected to live-in. Essentially, this was to be with the child at all times. A father explained this moral dimension clearly when he spoke critically of how some parents 'treated the nurses':

> We sit here all week and we're here every day, you know, so she always has either me or her mother here, but there's other folk in the ward will just walk away, they'll put their bairn to sleep and come back three hours later (. . .) sometimes I think they think it's a kinda holiday camp. (12, p. 2)

This account illustrated another important pressure which parents felt, the judgement of other parents. This father made what he believed to be a good case for his and his wife's moral adequacy as good live-in parents. They were not only present in the ward every day but they were always sitting right beside their child's bed. The sense of moral obligation which parents described had another dimension, that of the repayment of a privilege. Both nurses and parents were aware of the negative comments that some parents could attract were they not to demonstrate a visible caring commitment towards their child. The impression gained from the interviews was that parents perceived living-in with their child as a privilege which they had been afforded. Thus they were fortunate to be allowed to live-in as opposed to the ward staff being fortunate that parents were able and willing to live-in. Where parents perceived living-in in this way, it is understandable that they then felt under obligation to repay or earn this privilege by trying to be a 'good parent' according to what they believed to be the values of the hospital and ward. While being constantly there with and for your child was one way of repaying, the other was to try to be as helpful to ward staff as possible. As one parent explained:

> I think you feel as though you're privileged that you've been allowed to stay in with them, so you do as much as possible for them so maybe the nurses think, oh, thank Christ she's in here! (26, Mother 5, p. 90)

3.1.2 Being guilty

Parental guilt has been reported as a pervasive accompanying feature of accidents and illness among children. However, this guilt has been viewed predominantly as part of a more diffuse anxiety pattern or crisis reaction to hospitalization (Eltzer, 1984) and has not been specifically linked to the moral dimension of being a live-in parent.

While some parents were able to accept that their child's injury or illness was a genuine accident or due to circumstances outwith their direct control, it was more common for parents to describe how they blamed themselves. Parents blamed themselves for their child's injury and punished themselves for 'allowing' the accident to happen. For the parents of burned children there was another 'dread-full' pang to their guilt. This was their omnipresent fear of any future disfigurement and scarring that the child might suffer. Had the child 'only' broken a leg as a result of the accident, this could heal invisibly. With a burn or scald, however, the child's scarring would be a permanent, visible accusation of the parent's failure in that most primordial area of being a parent, protecting your child. In this respect, nurses' moral judgements as to whether parents were responsible for, or had somehow caused or contributed to their child's injury were significant in determining parents' moral standing within the ward. I shall return to this point in the latter section of this chapter.

An important influence in the shaping of parents' moral identities was the obligation which was placed upon them to show that they were 'competent' parents. Parents whose child had been injured in an accident often had their competence as parents called into question, especially in Ward B, the burns unit. These parents seemed to feel more obliged than others to re-establish their moral identities as good parents by showing that they were, after all, still competent to care for their child.

As with many of the burns and scalds, the fact that the child's accident occurred in the home seemed to accentuate the guilt that parents experienced. The home is a powerful metaphor for family care and safety which gives accidents which occur here an additional dimension of parental blameworthiness which is less apparent than in those where the child is perhaps playing outside with friends. When such accidents occurred parents were highly critical of their own competence, feeling that they had caused the accident to occur and that they had failed to protect their child. These parents' feelings were widely shared:

> It must have been my fault . . . how could I have been **so stupid**. . . . I was sure that I'd put the kettle far enough back. (. . .) Why did I do it? and **why** didn't I just think that the kettle was actually there? (10, p. 5)

> I think I just blame myself for what happened to him . . . and everybody keeps saying it was an accident, but I just can't get that into my head, I just blame myself for it . . . if I'd been . . . I only went through for a towel, if I'd been there it wouldn't have happened. (25, Mother 2, p. 48)

The guilt experienced by parents was not exclusively restricted to parents whose children had been injured in accidents. Parents whose children developed an illness could equally feel that they were somehow to blame, for example, for not noticing sooner that something was wrong with their child and for not seeking medical help earlier. One mother described how she felt that she might have 'allowed' her baby to develop severe breathing difficulties:

> I started to think (. . .) I must just be the worst mother that has ever been, because I haven't noticed my baby struggling [for breath]. (17, p. 16)

Parents wanted to be with their child and tried to ensure that they were there beside the child's bed during their waking hours and often even while their child slept. However, parents quickly gained the impression that this was also an expectation held by staff. This combination of choice and perceived pressure existed to the extent that parents felt guilty if, for example they left the ward to go for a tea or coffee break. As one father observed:

> They make you . . . well you feel guilty if you go away for a fag, you know . . . if you go away for a break you feel guilty. (25, Father 3, p. 6–7)

Parents were acutely sensitive to nurses' expressions of overt disapproval at their leaving the bedside. They also sensed more subtle hints which suggested that while such leaving might be tolerable, it was not actively encouraged by nurses. One parent spoke of one of the more obvious non-verbal ways in which nurses could convey such impressions:

> I think it's just the **looks** that you get (. . .) I'm frightened to go away in case they think 'You're not wanting anything to do with that bairn'. (25, Mother 2, p. 12)

Although no nurse was said to have stated explicitly that she disapproved of parents leaving their child's bedside, parents would occasionally detect supposedly humorous remarks which were more barbed than witty. For example, a father described how, while he was with a nurse who was bathing his son, his wife had returned to the ward with another child's mother [the two mothers having been for coffee together]:

> Jason was in the bath and my wife was out with Lindsay's mum. . . . My wife had come back and Nurse Pink had come in and says, 'Oh there's Mrs Jones back from her gallivanting'. (18, p. 41)

This was a telling remark as it highlighted how nurses seemed to differentiate between legitimate and illegitimate parental absences from the ward. Leaving the ward for a tea or coffee break or for lunch was seen as legitimate. This could be frowned upon, though, if the parent's timing was wrong and consequently a nurse was obliged to feed or change their child while they were away. Similarly, one mother whose child had been unsettled in the early part of the morning was 'ticked off' for absenting herself prior to a doctors' morning round:

> It was about ten to nine before we left and we said to Nurse Stone, 'We're just going for our breakfast,' . . . and she said, 'Well, you'll miss the doctors coming round . . . **you'll miss the doctors**' . . . well, you only get to half past nine for your breakfast! (25, Mother 1, p. 11)

Nurses also commented on how long the parents had been away for meals and breaks or, in a response which inevitably increased parents' guilt, they would report that their child had been crying for them or had 'needed them' during their absence.

It was not only the comments or actions of nurses which could increase parents' sense of guilt. Parents were also very aware that they could be equally critically judged by other parents. They described how they judged the care that other parents gave their children. They were also acutely aware of children who did not receive regular visitors and who they deemed to be 'just abandoned'. A group of parents speaking of a particular baby in the ward, described their critical reactions to other parents who 'left their children':

> **Mother 4:** He's been in two weeks and **nobody's** been in to see him . . . and I could take him home in a minute.
> **Mother 2:** Well, honestly, I could say for that baby, why is the mother not visiting him? It's not possible all the time for a mother to stay, some have two young children at home. . . .
> **Mother 3:** They could make an effort to visit.
> **Mother 2:** . . . but somebody could be there.
> **Mother 4: Nobody's** been there. . . . I don't judge the parents who come in but I judge the parents who don't come in at all. (26, p. 73–74)

The impression given by parents and indeed by nurses was that there was a moral continuum of parental 'goodness', based upon the amount and the nature of the time that parents spent with their hospitalized child.

This need to keep vigil beside the child was so strongly felt by some parents that one parent felt that it was somehow improper that she should be having such enjoyment, in the form of a coffee break, while her child remained seriously ill in the ward:

> Well, with Lucy being as she is now, all I can think about is that she is sat there and nothing is happening to her, so while I'm in here [the parents' sitting room/coffee room] enjoying my drink and my cigarette she's sat there gazing into space (. . .) you know, you feel so guilty because you're not there. (4, p. 14)

I have previously shown that parents who lived-in decided this virtually automatically. This was not a decision which required them to have goals, objectives or a clear sense of purpose. They were parents whose place was with their child, especially at this time. However, from the parents' accounts, it became clear that they came to feel a need to establish a moral purpose to their living-in. They also had to decide how they were going to approach the everyday business of being a live-in parent in such a way that they could re-establish their moral identity as a good parent, especially if the circumstances of the child's admission had fractured this image. I now explore the ways in which parents tried to establish or re-establish their moral identity.

3.2 ESTABLISHING AND RE-ESTABLISHING MORAL IDENTITIES

Parents described several approaches and strategies which they used in order to establish their moral identity as a 'good parent'. These approaches were geared towards being useful and were characterized by compliance and a seeming attempt on the part of parents to appear as helpful as possible and to avoid being seen as demanding or a nuisance.

3.2.1 Defensive parenting: being 'in the presence of experts'

Parents tried to establish their moral adequacy through what I term 'defensive parenting'. This was a strategy which parents adopted in order to better approximate the practices and therefore the perceived 'goodness' of nursing staff. The underlying basis of this strategy seemed to be the belief that nurses practised a more acceptable form of child care within the context of the ward and that this was a style or approach which parents should emulate. I introduced this idea in Chapter 2 in the discussion of parents' and nurses' respective disciplinary ethos but here I stress the implications of such discrepant perspectives for parents' moral status.

Parents' accounts suggested that they perceived an idealized way of caring for the child which was exemplified in the nurses' practices. In contrast, the parents' child-care practices were therefore considered less legitimate within the moral context of the ward. One mother described this in relation to her pre-adolescent daughter who was semi-comatose following a severe head injury and who had to have a nappy [diaper] changed regularly:

> You know there's things that you say, 'I must do this' or 'I must get this right' . . . things like when you're changing her . . . you change her the way the nurses change her rather than the way you would if you was at home doing it. You wouldn't, sort of, spend five minutes saying 'Come on, lift your bottom up', you'd go, 'Oh never mind that', up the knees would go and that would be it, but you know that somebody else is watching you or you think they are, so you've got to, sort of, make your patience go longer. (4, p. 25–26)

It would be understandable for parents to feel uncertain of their own child-care abilities in areas which might be defined as being more technical or medical. What is especially significant here is that parents seemed to recognize the moral superiority of nurses' expertise and practices even in areas of care so 'basic' as changing a child's nappy. Strong (1979a) has shown that the professional assumption regarding an idealized vision of parental competence 'was potentially undercut by the most routine of medical practices' (Strong, 1979a, p. 163). Silverman (1987) has also argued, and I agree, that when parents' perceived functions and responsibilities are passed to 'experts', the parents' sense of moral responsibility and competence is threatened. I would extend the argument, however, to suggest that it is not only when the responsibility and the tasks are transferred that parents feel threatened. Parents in this study felt similarly threatened when the criteria for determining the quality of their child care were set and controlled not by themselves but by professionals. This was made clear in a dialogue between two mothers during a focus group interview:

> **Mother 1:** It's because you feel in the presence of experts that will disapprove of your inadequacies.
> **Mother 2:** They've been trained how to feed and change a baby, whereas you just . . . (26, p. 46)

These parental perceptions seemed to be particularly characteristic of the early stage of the parents' stay in hospital. As parents became more familiar with the ward and hospital and as they developed strategies and approaches to help them deal with situations, they became more comfortable with this aspect of living-in. As one mother explained:

> At the beginning, yeah, 'Am I doing the right things?' 'Am I washing her properly?' (laughs) . . . and sort of silly things like that . . . but now I just think . . . it doesn't bother me now 'cos I've got used to it, but at first you're very conscious. (10, p. 57)

3.2.2 Showing an interest

Nurses formed much of their assessment of parents' moral identities from what they observed of their behaviour. As these nurses explained, it was important that parents showed clearly recognizable affection and caring in their interactions with the child and also that they were 'appropriately' upset regarding the child's illness or injury:

> **Nurse A:** I think we expect them to show, if they're living in, to show face and to be in the ward a lot. . . .
> **Nurse B:** And show great concern.
> **Nurse A:** I think just show face, show concern and comfort the child. (20, p. 46)

An important element of 'showing an interest' was that good parents were expected to be inquisitive and to have a keen interest in their child's condition and treatment. However for parents, this posed a real dilemma. While they were interested to the point of preoccupation in their child's condition, they had to perform a difficult social and moral balancing act as they strove to find out information.

For parents, finding out was not simply a matter of having a question or query and then asking a nurse or doctor for an answer. Information-seeking called for a delicate social balancing which parents had to accomplish if they were to establish themselves as concerned and interested while avoiding appearing to be 'a nuisance' or 'neurotic'. To be successful at finding out in both informational and moral terms required a carefully considered approach on the part of parents, an approach which was usually based upon unfailing courtesy and politeness (cf. Strong, 1979a; Silverman, 1987; Robbins and Wolf, 1988).

Parents were aware that, unless they requested information in a particular way, they ran the risk of being labelled as 'silly', 'over-anxious', 'neurotic' or simply 'a nuisance', which would in turn lead to their receiving even less information and also damaging their moral identity. It was very important therefore for parents to think carefully not only about what they wished to ask but also about whom they would ask and how they would ask. This mother explained this very well:

> I find I have to sort of think, am I choosing the right time to go and speak to them, otherwise they'll be saying, 'Well I've got to go and do a drip or I've got to do this now' or . . . I sort of watch them and see what they're doing and try to catch them at a moment when I know they're either just walking up to the kitchen or going to the linen room or something, so that you feel that you're not stopping them from doing anything that's vital. (. . .) I think what I'm going to ask and I try to ask in as nice a way as possible (. . .) asking if something's possible or if it's all right to do something, rather ask their permission even if it is for something that's there. Normally they'd say, 'Well, go and help yourself', but I'd rather ask so that you're on the right side, really. (2, p. 29)

The importance of approach and manner for parents went beyond commonplace politeness and courtesy. There was a shared perception among parents that a carefully considered approach was essential to prevent them from 'getting on the wrong side' of the staff thus making their situation worse (cf. Robinson, 1985). This wrong side was not inhabited by good parents who were concerned for their child, caring, helpful, interested and polite. On the wrong side were parents who were 'neurotic', 'nuisances', 'nosy', or 'thick'. Being excluded from the moral community of good parents in this way had uncomfortable implications for the parents themselves but there was a more worrying prospect. This was expressed by parents who felt that their child was hostage to their performance as good parents. Parents believed that somehow, their child's care and indeed the child could suffer as a result of any of their actions which might place them on the 'wrong side' of staff.

3.2.3 Avoiding social activities

Nurses generally expected parents to avoid any social activities or overt displays of enjoyment. Each nurse seemed to have their own particular favourite story, not unlike contemporary 'urban legends' (Brunvand, 1981; 1984), and professional 'atrocity stories' (Dingwall, 1977; Baruch, 1981). These described parents who were felt to have misused their time in the hospital by having fun instead of being with their child. These narratives would often concern either individuals or perhaps a group of parents who held a wild party in the Mothers' Unit. One nurse described her experience with one such set of parents:

> We had an older girl that was in as well and her mum and sort of boyfriend had come down and they ended up not staying in the hostel but with friends nearby . . . so they could come in to see her [the child], or they came in and it was actually pathetic, if the man hadn't made the excuses, it would have been better than . . . 'We had trouble this morning with the car 'cos the roads were really busy' and they were about three hours late and you think, shut up!, don't lie, don't bother, just be honest . . . (mimics parent's 'feigned concern' voice) 'Hello, Annie. How are you doing, love?' Very nicey nicey and the coats weren't even off and they were away again . . . and you think why upset her by coming in for such a short time and what the hell are you going to be doing for the rest of the day, kind of thing, that is annoying. (. . .) It was a waste of time, and it was obvious that they just wanted a room to themselves somewhere, that they could have a bit of fun, basically, and that was sussed out immediately. (16, p. 56–57)

Another nurse told of a 'Mothers' Unit party':

> We had a mum who came to live-in and only stayed two nights then just didn't want to live-in any more and nobody could figure out why, 'cos this had been planned, that she would live-in . . . and it turned out that she'd

been sharing a room with a mother who'd been having parties till three o'clock in the morning in the room and the room was like a pigsty and this girl just couldn't live like that. But nobody . . . . . . again it was, 'Why doesn't this mother want to stay in?' . . . and it was her who was condemned because she was the one who left . . . police and things were called in that incident as well. (29, Nurse 1, p. 20)

The nurses' expectation that good parents would abstain from social activities and devote their attention to their child was revealed clearly during the period of fieldwork in the burn's unit. One live-in mother whose toddler had been in the ward for over two months had begun to regularly visit a local pub in the evenings and had actually joined their darts team. She had also taken to going for walks in a nearby park where she had befriended a woman who lived close to the hospital and had subsequently been regularly invited to this woman's house for meals.

The reaction of most of the nursing staff, and indeed of the other ward parents, to this parent's social activities was extremely hostile and critical. It was openly expressed that this mother was neglecting her primary responsibility to her child, abusing the privilege of being allowed a room in the Mothers' Unit and generally, in a popular phrase, 'treating the place like a holiday camp'.

From my conversations with the mother, however, a different interpretation emerged. She felt that as a young mother she had already spent a very long time as a virtual 'in-patient' in the hospital and therefore deserved to get out to socialize. She also made the point that she was an isolated young mother whose marriage had been traumatic, often brutal and probably about to end soon. This was, for her, a chance to make some new friends and psychologically 're-charge her batteries' during what was a long hospitalization.

Socializing while living-in was not invariably damaging to parents' moral standing. The key mediating factor seemed to be whether the socializing had violated the control norms of the ward, that is, whether the parents were socializing with or without staff permission. Nurses often said to parents who had been living-in for some time that they should try to get out for an occasional meal or drink together. This, however, was nurse-initiated and controlled and was usually suggested for the express purpose of allowing the parents to 'have a bit of a break'. There was no intent to encourage parents to establish any potentially regular or close contacts or interests which would possibly distract them from their primary responsibility, the child.

3.2.4 Pulling your weight

A parent's moral identity was threatened if their willingness to work as a live-in parent was called into question and strengthened if their helpfulness was obvious. The main component of their work while in hospital was the direct basic mothering related to their child's physical care. Parents were clearly aware that this was predominantly their responsibility. As this mother noted:

I don't think anything was said. (. . .) I think it's just expected that if a parent's there, they'll do things. (2, p. 43)

This expectation seemed greater when the child was perceived as being less seriously ill than other children in the ward. In such circumstances the tacit understanding was that parents would take over more of the child's care. The nurses could then work with more dependent children. As one mother remarked:

Aye, the better your child gets, the more well they get, the less attention they get. (27,Mrs B, p. 57)

Another mother described how, in a previous experience of living-in in a different hospital, she had felt this pressure to carry out her parental work:

This particular night I was completely shattered and all I wanted to do was go to my bed (. . .) he was to be fed at midnight and I really didn't want to stay up to do it and I said, 'Will somebody be able to feed him at midnight?' . . . and they said, 'Oh well, we're a bit pushed, could you not just stay up and do it?' . . . and I couldn't say no, I couldn't say, 'No!, I'm going to my bed!' . . . 'cos I felt so guilty, and I felt really guilty for asking (. . .) they just made me feel guilty, because I wanted to go away to my bed and there were other babies there who were sicker than mine. . . . (17, p. 28–29)

Parents' sense of moral identity was closely entwined with their feelings of self-confidence and of competence as caregivers to their child. Their perceptions of themselves as good parents could therefore be diminished if they had no clear sense of exactly how they were to translate their concern for the child's well-being and desire to be there with them into the more instrumental and functional activities which they felt were expected of them.

This was highlighted particularly in the cases of the children who had suffered serious head injuries and were minimally responsive to their surroundings. Their parents expressed deep frustration and anger at having no clear idea as to how they as parents were expected to help in the child's recovery. A mother who stayed in the ward during the day with her daughter explained that she felt:

very guilty because you can't do anything when you are here, but when you're away you want to be back here. (4, p. 5)

Parents were expected to demonstrate their competence and worth by being active participants in the basic care of their child, depending upon the seriousness of the child's illness or injury. To determine the origins of such expectations it is useful to examine the ways in which the nurses explained the value of having resident parents in the ward. For such explanations were notable for their almost exclusive concentration upon how participating parents were a help to nurses, especially when they were particularly busy. Several nurses explained this:

I think they are valued for what they do, 'cos I remember some shifts when you couldn't function without parents there . . . you know, there's just not enough staff. I remember one evening being on with a first-year nurse, just the two of us . . . and the ward was full and if there hadn't been parents there we'd be still trying to feed all of them now (laughs) . . . we just wouldn't have managed. (Nurse B, 29, p. 14)

Oh, especially when you are busy, feeding them and that . . . things that take up quite a bit of time when you are busy, especially. (. . .) When you're busy I think really that you value them more than anything. (23, p. 6)

It gives you free time to do other things, basically. If the child's upset, Mum can go and comfort it . . . you don't have to sit there for an hour or what-ever and nurse the child when you don't have the time 'cos you've got a list of other things to do. (29, p. 13)

These nurses' accounts revealed that participation might not have been seen as a genuine collaborative and sharing arrangement between nurse and parent regarding all aspects of the child's hospitalization and care. Rather, it might have been one where the good parent was seen as being synonymous with the good ward helper. This helper's value increased with their willingness to pull their weight, especially where they displayed this willingness during times of staffing shortages or very high workload.

3.2.5 Not being a nuisance

In order to be seen as a willing worker, it was important for parents that they did not spoil this by creating the impression of being a nuisance in the eyes of the nurses. The importance of this perception became clear as the parents' accounts frequently described how busy the nurses were. In such circumstances it is clear to see how parental interruptions were thought to be unwelcome.

I don't interrupt **anybody**, **ever**. I interrupt people as little as possible. (6, p. 12)

Another reason for parents' reluctance to be a nuisance by making too many demands upon nurses was that they often perceived other children in the ward to be more in need of the nurses' attentions than their child. Thus in making demands or requests they were depriving more deserving cases of the nursing attention that was more appropriately theirs. One mother whose son had been admitted for a waiting-list hypospadias repair put this particularly well:

You feel guilty 'cos, oh there's nothing really wrong with my kid and there's other kids really ill, and here's me complaining. (13, p. 24)

This feeling was not expressed solely by parents of children who were less seri-ously ill, for example, those who had been admitted for waiting-list surgery or routine investigations. The mother of one of the children who had suffered a very severe head injury as the result of a road traffic accident, noted that

> although you think your kid's bad, there's always somebody else worse. (5, p. 27–28)

Parents felt uncomfortable about making requests and demands of nurses, especially if these were unusual, in the sense that they were time-consuming or disruptive of the ward routine. One mother described how she had found it difficult to ask if her toddler could be moved to another ward or area as the ward was so busy and noisy that he could not get to sleep:

> but I hate making a stir anyway 'cos I get myself – this is terrible – I felt I was all tied up in a knot . . . well, I wanted to do something but I didn't want to make a fuss. (2, p. 15–16)

In this discussion of the ways in which parents attempted to establish their moral identities as good parents, I have argued that their strategies were essentially those which reflected and maintained their subservient position within the ward. When parents were unsure of how to be a live-in parent or exactly what was expected of them, it seemed that they tried, at least initially, to adapt their parenting and practices to what they perceived to be the prevailing orthodoxy of the ward. The pressures to conform in this way helped to shape the parents' perceptions that to do otherwise would threaten their moral identity and make them more of a nuisance than a good parent.

3.2.6 Being competent

The accounts of both parents and nurses suggested that a tension existed between the parents' practical, particular and personal knowledge of their child and the nurses' general professional knowledge of paediatrics. Parents expressed the view that nurses had an expertise which demanded recognition by virtue of their professional training and as the discussion of defensive parenting showed, they would often modify their usual parenting style in deference to nurses' professional child care approaches.

In the area of 'basic mothering' parents might have been expected to feel more confident of their own specific practices because these were such integral parts of their and their child's lives. But as I will show, the moral sense of such 'basic mothering' tasks changed for parents within the alien world of the ward.

Parents' confidence in their ability to provide their child's care in the ward could be shaken when their competence was called into question by hospital staff. But such questioning, either subtle or explicit, of competence also represented a challenge to the parents' sense of self. One mother described this in relation to an incident where a nurse had suggested that her toddler son would take his lunch better if she left the ward while a nurse fed the child:

... it was like the other day, we got told to go away so they could get food into him. ... We felt terrible 'cos we had to go away, felt as if we weren't feeding him right, you know. ... (25, Mother 2, p. 67)

This was a fairly clear strategy which left the mother in little doubt that both her competence and moral standing as a good mother were in question. Other, more subtle ways in which parents' competence could be called into question included what one mother has previously described as 'the look' of withering disapproval. Another mother described the unspoken disapproval that she had received when she initially seemed unwilling to carry out certain aspects of her child's care:

I was really frightened to touch him ... because the nurse knew how to handle him, 'cos he'd been burnt ... and there was a few times I would say, 'Look, could you maybe change his bum or could you give him a wash, could you do this ... I'm frightened.' And they were looking at me as if to say, ... 'Well, you're his mum, are you that [so] stupid you don't know what to do?' (15, p. 33)

This was a particularly good illustration of the point that what was at home the simplest of routine tasks was now infused with fear, uncertainty and complexity. However, for the nurses concerned, this was still considered to be a simple, routine and mundane task. These discrepant perspectives created a situation where the mother's reluctance could be interpreted not as tiredness, fear or uncertainty but as evidence that the mother was lazy, stupid or unwilling to help out. Overt questioning of a parent's moral status as a good mother was rare. However, this particular mother did have her moral adequacy questioned in a much more official and explicit manner, as was shown in Chapter 2's discussion of parents and discipline.

Parents also felt that their competence was being undermined when their understandings or perspectives were disregarded or belittled by hospital staff. One mother expressed a common viewpoint when she said that

One of the things that really annoys me is when you're asked your opinion ... not your opinion but you're asked about something and say whatever it is and think, they're not believing a word I'm saying, they're taking no notice of what I'm saying. (13, p. 20)

When the professional explanation conflicted with a parent's account of events there was a knowledge value differential weighted against the parent. One mother whose baby had severe respiratory difficulties described this process of losing confidence in her knowledge of her own child:

I really started to question my judgement, because all the doctors kept asking me if he had been perfectly healthy before, and he had been and he'd had all his regular check-ups (. . .) but I started (. . .) the more people started asking me the question 'Was he perfectly all right?', in **my mind** implying

that he couldn't **possibly** have been, I started to think, I haven't noticed this
. . . and my judgement counts for nothing. (17, p. 15–16)

Parents had vivid recollections of occasions when their knowledge of their child
was disregarded or disbelieved by doctors or nurses. One mother described such
an incident when her daughter developed an infection:

> She was awful whingy, she was awful listless and her tummy was making
> awful grumbling noises . . . so I says to a few nurses, but there was no atten-
> tion taken at the time, so from eight o'clock to 12 that night my daughter's
> breathing went from regular to hardly any at all. I lifted her eyelids, her
> pupils were pinpointed, she was floppy (. . .) so I says to the nurse . . . she
> says 'But that's her [she's just] in a deep sleep', I says, 'She's not, her
> breathing's not right, her eyes are pinpointed.' I says, 'I'm not happy with
> her and I'm not moving till I get a doctor in to see her' . . . so she went and
> got another nurse and she went and got another nurse (. . .) so the end result
> was the Sister came up and she looked at her and says, 'You're right, there
> is something wrong', then a Registrar came down. (5, p. 38–39)

It is possible that in situations such as this, where the child's medical condition
was the prime focus of professional attention, parental knowledge was seen to be
at its least reliable and relevant. The parent was in the position of trying to participate in an arena of discourse where professional knowledge and professional
language were the accepted currency.

3.3 NURSES AND PARENTS' MORAL IDENTITIES

I suggested in Chapter 2 that the nurses had clear expectations of live-in parents,
for example that they should be co-operative, competent and of good character.
This latter point supports the arguments that 'parenting is a moral issue' (Baruch,
1981, p. 292) and that a parent's identity is not only socially but morally constituted (Gubrium and Buckholdt, 1982a). This section discusses the ways in which
nurses helped to shape parents' moral identities.

3.3.1 Creating parents' moral identities

This was illustrated in the following nurse's lengthy account. I was aware from
my conversations with this nurse and with other ward staff that a particular
mother in the ward was giving the staff cause for concern and 'causing problems'. I asked the nurse how she thought this mother was seen by the staff and
this general opening prompted an extremely detailed 18-page description of how
the nurse viewed this particular parent and of the problems that she posed for the
staff. Embedded within this lengthy account were indications of the ways in
which the moral and social sense of parenthood was created:

As a live-in parent she was seen . . . you see she went through all the different stages that I'm sure . . . like, she was 19 years old for a kick off and . . . . . . being away from home . . . she went. . . . At the very beginning we used to encourage her to go back home to be with Susan, the wee one, just for bonding purposes and things like that, and then she went home for a couple of days, then we sort of realized that she didn't want to go home. She likes it better here 'cos she's got the social life here, and it was ages and ages before anything was done about that. And I think that was to her cost in a way, 'cos I don't think she was awful happy doing what she was doing . . . and she didn't have the maturity to realize that what was happening was affecting her relationship with her wee boy, 'cos she was never here, and also her daughter at home, the baby, 'cos she was never there . . . and she was just more or less having a wee holiday camp time here . . . and I think it upset her 'cos she was living in the Mothers' Unit, she was out and about with men, etcetera, . . . I mean, this is an extreme example, they're not all like this . . . and I think it's a perfect example of an unhappy lady, who is trying to enjoy the freedom but can't . . . and she had nobody to say, 'Can't do it, Mary, stay in here and look after your wee boy.' (16, p. 33–34)

The nurse immediately mentioned that this mother was very young with two children, '19 years old for a kick off', and 'didn't have the maturity to realize what was happening'. The mother's age seemed to be important in helping to construct her as not a 'proper' parent, to the extent that, even at the outset, the nurses felt that they needed to help her achieve 'bonding' with her other child at home. She had also contravened another unwritten tenet of proper parenthood when she seemed to put her own enjoyment before the needs of her child by going out of the hospital to social functions. This made the nurses feel, as another nurse described to me, that they were 'built-in free baby-sitters'. The nurse felt that this mother had failed to fulfil the expectations of proper parenthood by not being there for her child, both in the phenomenological and more practical sense of being available to help with his care at the busy times, for example mealtimes and early morning. The nurse also highlighted another factor in the social and moral creation of proper parenthood when she suggested that the mother's sexual relationships were questionable.

When she wasn't here – see, this is where the gossip from the other mothers start – she was sharing a room with another mother and . . . her room was seemingly filthy, she was never in it, and then when she was she had a man in it, at least one man in it, and this isn't just idle gossip, this is known fact. (16, p. 38)

That she was said to have been 'out and about with men' was taken by nurses as further indication of her lack of claim to proper parenthood. Interestingly, this nurse suggested that proper parents could not expect to have this degree of freedom while living-in in hospital because all must be secondary to staying in and looking after your child. Should parents fail to live-in within this constraint, the result was surely be their and their child's unhappiness. The nurse described what she called 'sensible parents' and explained how this mother was seen as being a 'non sensible parent':

> I think that the situation was really difficult because she was a **non-sensible** mum in the eyes of Mr Purple [a Consultant] say, for example, 'cos he was of the opinion that if this child went home, OK, Granny was a sort of strict type and would make sure the wee boy was properly looked after, all that sort of thing (. . .) we thought Gran could cope at home, 'cos she is, she's very good. (16, p. 41)

This mother was now additionally cast as lacking in the competence needed to care for her child. It seemed as if this proper parenthood was shifted on to the grandmother, who was then seen as effectively more of a real parent than the mother herself. The factors which contributed to the moral and social construction of proper parenthood by nurses were not mutually exclusive and were often blurred. For example, in explaining why this mother was not seen as a 'sensible mother', the nurse described both the social conditions that led to the attribution of this label and the moral dimension of these social features:

> **PD:** Two things there, one . . . that she was not seen as a sensible [mother] . . .
> **Nurse:** Yes, that's right.
> **PD:** Why not?
> **Nurse:** Well, for example, just the fact that there was a social worker involved at home anyway, Dad was a heroin addict, separated . . . in here, there was an incident in here when Dad came in drunk or stoned or high one night, and he had started to shout about the place and he was annoyed 'cos Wendy wasn't here, she said she was by the bedside and she was away out, you know . . . whatever . . . she actually she got in a darts team here as well, she used to go out and play some evenings . . . and it was – Philip, it was just sort of a social thing for her, it was like a nine-to-five for her. . . . She didn't have the hassle of looking after the baby, she never had the hassle of looking after him, so it was just a sort of all day thing and she coped quite nicely with that, thank you very much, you know . . . and it was a very difficult situation. (16, p. 42–43)

This mother, it seemed, had abdicated not only her parental role and responsibilities in favour of an easier and more enjoyable form of living-in, but had also given up with them the possibility of being seen as a proper and 'sensible' parent. Gubrium and Buckholdt (1982a) stress that the social and moral constitution of family is not of purely theoretical interest. Here, the nurses' accounts of what they deemed to be difficult parents or families were instructive. Nurses felt that it was very difficult for them to talk to or to relate to parents and families when they did not behave in the ways that nurses believed that families should. Such behaviour would prompt what Gubrium and Buckholdt (1982a) refer to as 'What kind of family is this?' type of questioning. For example, the nurse cited previously felt unable to 'get involved' in this mother's family because they were constituted in terms of social problems and 'wrangles':

> It was all very difficult, 'cos it wasn't up to us to get involved in that either [the grandmother had apparently been phoning the ward and had been unable to locate the mother], you know, the sort of family wrangle thing. (16, p. 49)

Similarly, when parents refused to accept what was felt to be the reasonable advice of the nurse, it became difficult for the nurse to develop any sort of dialogue or relationship. This nurse described how she had tried to advise the mother against giving her toddler Chinese food as it was felt that this had made him 'severely hyperactive' and had caused other problems:

> And I said, 'and the prawn crackers gave him diarrhoea last time', and she said, '**Oh, no**, if I want to slip him a prawn cracker I'll slip him a prawn cracker,' and I said, 'Fine!' You can only say so much, you can't dictate to them what they have to do. (16, p. 50–51)

Another nurse described a situation where a parent's 'obnoxious' behaviour was seen as being so alien to that expected from a proper parent that the nurse was unable to relate to him on even a basic conversational level:

> I just feel that when you get situations like that it tends to be definitely the personality of the person, 'cos another situation with Kevin, who's actually dying and the father is so obnoxious to the extent that the child's terminally ill at home, the mother phoned up and asked if the doctor could come out and visit at home 'cos they were worried . . . and they went out and the father was more interested in the football on the telly than talking to the doctor . . . you know, he's just that sort of person, a little nyaff [good-for-nothing] (laughs) and, I mean, it's **really hard** to talk to that man . . . and be pleasant to him when you know he's not in the slightest bit interested and he's such an **obnoxious** person . . . and you think, I just don't want to talk to him. I wouldn't go near the man, basically . . . I'll talk to his wife but . . . it got to the stage where I just couldn't even look at him he just made me so angry. (31, Nurse C, p. 33–34)

3.3.2 Judging the judgers?

One approach to an examination of the nurses' assessments, expectations and perceptions of parents would be to regard the nurses' accounts as evidence of professional dominance and labelling. Parents had certain characteristics and behaviours which the nurses either approved or disapproved of, valued or did not value and tolerated or did not tolerate. Consequently, the nurses seemed open to accusations of exerting professional dominance over the parents or of making unsubstantiated moral judgements. Kelly and May's (1982) criticisms of this approach are both timely and apposite: 'A high moral tone pervades the literature in the sense that serious professional weaknesses and deficiencies have been identified, namely that some patients receive better treatment than others because some are labelled good and some are labelled bad' and 'Few of the researchers have considered the possibility that the reason for some patients being defined as bad is not because staff are inadequately trained or are unprofessional, but because bad patients do in fact make nursing and medical staff's life difficult (Kelly and May, 1982, p. 152).

If these nurses' accounts were abstracted from their context, they could be taken as evidence for the claim that nurses made premature and uninformed judgements regarding parents, and that they based such judgements upon professionally questionable concepts such as the parent's intelligence, personality and general demeanour. In this way the nurses could be rendered open to both professional and personal criticism. There are several reasons why I avoided such an approach in this study.

The impression gained from the nurses' accounts was that they were uncomfortable with and hesitant in their use of the terms 'intelligence' and 'personality' as they applied these to parents. I sensed a recognition that these terms did not adequately capture what they wished to convey regarding how they used their clinical knowledge and experience to reach understandings of parents.

Nurses' assessments affected the parents' stay in hospital and the nature of their subsequent involvement in the child's care. Yet it seemed that the nurses did not have an adequate discourse of engagement which would allow them to discuss how they would help parents to become genuinely involved in the care of their child. This may partly explain the lack of dialogue which existed between parents and nurses regarding the nature of parents' future involvement in their child's care during their stay in hospital.

The nurses needed to ascertain whether the parents were willing to help or whether they were apprehensive about participation and about their child's stay in hospital in general. They also had to try to determine whether the parents would be able to carry out any care competently and safely as they believed that it was nurses who were ultimately legally and professionally responsible for the child.

Nurses' initial assessments of parents seemed brief and superficial. The first impressions that nurses developed were formed during times, such as the child's admission, which were often hurried, especially if the child's admission was an emergency. It was also evident that nurses' perceptions of parents were influenced by the attitudes and expressed opinions of other nurses. It might be expected that such quick initial assessments would be supplemented and perhaps revised by more informed and reflective attempts at a future point during the parent's stay. While this seemed to occur on an individual basis with some nurses, where a nurse might change her mind about a parent, it did seem that initial impressions of parents were transmitted *ex cathedra* through the nursing system. Negative assessments of parents were difficult to alter. However, they could change positively when nurses approached parents from an involved, open, caring stance and where the conditions were such that nurses could have the kind of contact with the parents that was necessary to really 'get to know the person behind the parent', as one nurse expressed it.

In relation to the assessment of parents by neonatal unit staff, Bogdan *et al.* (1982, p. 11) argued that 'Most assessments of parents are based on limited knowledge, derived mainly from short observations, limited conversations or secondhand reporting of incidents and information. What is known is episodic, not informed by the context of the perinatal experience in the lives of the parents.'

Sosnowitz (1984), in another study of neonatal units, claimed that parent typologies such as 'emotionally fragile', 'hostile' and 'difficult parents as per chart' were routinely used by staff as assessments upon which future management decisions were made. However, these and other studies (Kelly and May, 1982) tended to see such first impressions as being fixed and unchanging. In contrast, the accounts of nurses in this research seemed to indicate that perceptions can alter both radically and positively, given the opportunity for sustained close and caring contact (see Benner, 1984; Benner and Wrubel, 1989). Critics of the way in which nurses make moral judgements concerning parents tend to ignore the fact that such reactions to people and events are almost universal human responses and not merely the manifestation of 'serious professional weaknesses' (Kelly and May, 1982).

Nurses are expected to be able to work with parents while being nonjudgemental unless, of course, such judgements are positive, in which case they are perfectly acceptable. If they are unable to achieve this then they are at least expected to be able to conceal any negative feelings which they might have regarding particular parents. In the absence of any forum or opportunities for nurses to discuss, vent and deal with such feelings, such as in a staff group (Beardslee and De Maso, 1982), they can build up and eventually spill over into other areas of the nurse's work or home life. One nurse described this:

> **Nurse:** You're trying to hide your feelings and hide your judgements, like you're walking about thinking these things and you bottle them all up and then all of a sudden you'll crack . . . and you crack up at each other.
> **PD:** Rather than at . . . ?
> **Nurse:** Rather than at the parents, 'cos at the moment there's a lot of feelings bottled up and there's a lot of feelings hidden from Sasha's mum, like . . . . . . and really we all feel the same, we all get really depressed about that and we take it all out on each other. (24, p. 30–31)

Another nurse described how the strain of hiding such illegitimate feelings had affected her relations at home and had eventually spilled out into an open display of 'coolness' towards Sasha's mother:

Nurse: I feel that, in a way, what she [Sasha's mother] did was wrong (. . .) but I try to forget that and try to be nice to her, you know, I don't feel bad towards her, really, no. . . .

PD: I suppose sometimes you must feel things towards people . . . but what do you do with it?

Nurse: I take it out on others (laughs). (. . .) I used to go home and take it out on my mother. (. . .) I was in here [the ICU] with Sasha and I'd come in and it was a bit of a guddle [mess] when I got in and it took a wee while to get organized and her mum was there. . . . I got myself organized, and then I dropped something on the floor and she said, 'It's not your night, is it?' the mum said to me, 'It's not your night, is it?' and I was so annoyed at her for saying that to me, you know, 'You've no right to say that sort of thing to me' . . . but I think she realized that she'd said something because I didn't speak to her for a wee while afterwards, you know. . . . (23, p. 12–14)

The nurses' accounts revealed tensions between themselves and live-in parents. Nurses stressed the individuality of parents and children and the importance for the nurse–parent relationship of the individual's personality. Yet the nurses also had to work within a framework where their concerns had to be both particular and universal. This was often expressed by nurses who described the difficulties involved in giving merited individual attention in a particular situation when they had 'another 20 children in the ward that need attention too'.

It seems as unrealistic to expect that nurses should never form opinions or make judgements of parents as it would be to expect parents never to judge nurses. Yet the nurses in this study gave the impression that they considered their judgements of parents to be illegitimate and almost unprofessional, especially if their judgements of a particular parent were negative.

3.3.3 Getting to know the person of the parent

Nurses' accounts suggested that parent's perceived moral adequacy was not always a fixed typological label such as 'neurotic parent' or 'negligent parent'. The case of one mother whose baby daughter was extensively scalded over her head, neck and face was particularly illustrative here and worth discussing at length.

I had been leaving some information leaflets about a future focus group meeting in the Mother's Unit when an extremely distraught mother was helped in by nurses and taken to her room. My first thought was that perhaps her child had just died. When I returned to the ward office I mentioned to a nurse what I had just seen. Also in the room was one of the hospital's senior nurses, who said, 'Well, it's a bit late to be distraught now!' and 'What do you expect when you leave a six-month-old baby unsupervised?' I was surprised at the vehemence of her comments, as I knew this nurse to be a caring and competent person and not usually given to such remarks.

It transpired that the mother whom I had seen in the Unit had a daughter who had been admitted to the ward with the most severe full-thickness facial scalds that many of the staff had ever seen. It was also clear that a climate of blame had quickly enveloped this mother, whose daughter's injuries were seen to be emphatically her fault. This feeling was fuelled when it was discovered that the mother's older child had also been hospitalized with a slight burn injury in the past. The mother had quickly been judged by the ward staff and found to have been negligent.

I wondered whether the prevalent judgement, that she was a criminally negligent mother, would be shared by the nurses as a group and whether such a judgement would be a fixed or changing concept. I also wondered, in such a climate of blame and criticism, who was going to 'be there' for this mother? Two nurses who had been involved in the baby's care discussed this during their interview when I asked if nurses tended to judge parents:

> You go on what you've been told, and when I first came to the ward they told the background to the case (. . .) they [judgements about parents] do get passed on, definitely. Most are at report time (. . .) people do form opinions and do pass them on to other people. (20, p. 34, 40)

This nurse's perceptions of the mother had been informed and influenced by another nurse:

> **PD:** What was the perception that you had before you knew her?'
> **Nurse A:** That she had another child who had been burned six months previously and this had happened and that it was sheer negligence, and was probably her fault and that it [her explanation for the incident] was all a story that she had fabricated to protect herself. That was the impression that I was given, from various members of staff, not least from one of the nurses on the Burns Course who was here the day Sasha was admitted and the girl was very angry about it and that was the impression she gave me. (. . .) She says, 'Wait till you go and see this kid, it's shocking what this mother's done to her', and then I came here and got told basically the same story from some of the staff . . . and you think, that's terrible, that's shocking, and you go in and you work with the woman . . . and you think . . . (shakes her head) (20, p. 41–42)

This nurse was regularly assigned to work with the baby and her mother in their cubicle, where her perceptions of this mother changed markedly:

> **Nurse A:** I went in and constant-cared Sasha and sat with her mother and I have nothing but respect for the woman now. . . . I don't lay a finger of blame at that woman's door and it's not for me to judge, but in my own mind I'm quite sure that she's not responsible for that injury and she shouldn't be made to suffer in the way that she has . . . no way. (20, p. 35)

There were two important issues here that I wanted to explore further. What had caused the nurse to revise her first impressions of Sasha's mother? and how had she felt that she had been 'made to suffer'? She described how staff who blamed Sasha's mother for her injuries made their disapproval of her known in ways which were often subtle and occasionally, less so:

PD: What do you mean, 'in the way she has?'
Nurse A: From [another nurse on the ward]'s attitude towards her on the ward, she's made to feel very guilty about what's happened to Sasha from her.
PD: How do you do that?
Nurse A: It's just her general (. . .) she says many things like . . . one wee scald we had, we were changing her dressings and she was crying and holding her arms out so that she [the nurse] could do the bandaging and she was going ma-ma-ma- and she says 'If your mama hadn't let you pull a cup of coffee over yourself this would never have bloody happened!' and I thought, you swine! and you know how many parents are sitting outside that treatment room door, and they hear . . . but she does that sort of thing in front of Sasha's mum all the time, she doesn't say anything directly to her but . . .
PD: It's within earshot?
Nurse A: Oh God, aye! (20, p. 36–37)

Having been presented with a negative and derogatory picture of this mother, Nurse A initially accepted these assessments but subsequently revised her perceptions:

That's what it's like, though, people do form opinions and pass them on to other people, but it's up to you whether you accept it as an individual . . . at first I did about this mum . . . Sasha's mum, and then, when I got to know her . . . (20, p. 41)

The nurse suggested that, while it seemed inevitable that nurses formed opinions and judgements of parents and discussed these among themselves, it was not equally inevitable that other nurses shared these and behaved accordingly towards the parent. The crucial factor here for this nurse was that she had the opportunity to 'get to know' this mother and to work closely with her and her baby. Mennerick (1974) has suggested that the use of client typologies will increase as the opportunity for worker–client interaction decreases. My interpretation would support such a claim while suggesting that the converse may also be the case. Nurse A described how her perceptions of this mother and her 'typification' as a negligent or bad mother had changed dramatically as a result of the nurse's being able to spend the time and have the human contact necessary in order to get to know the mother. When I asked how she had come to revise her thinking about this mother, the nurses explained.

Nurse B: Finding out the situation for yourself . . . reading the notes yourself . . . .

Nurse A: It wasn't even the notes, it was just speaking to her, 'cos she's just so ... upset and guilty and everything, and she doesn't know what's happening and she's got no perception of what Sasha's going to look like when she's older, and she's just so engulfed by that. You know she doesn't even care about the other two children now, she doesn't, she'll tell you that, she says the apple of my eye was Sasha and always will be, and the other two, I love them, but not like Sasha, and it's a damned sin 'cos her whole life is engulfed by this baby and I think it must be a real strain, their marriage must go through hell. I can imagine a lot of marriages breaking up through a child getting burned or injured where one parent is there and the other isn't, the strain they must go through is horrendous, I mean I've seen the two of them having stand-up fights in the ward, just snapping at each other and it's a damned shame. ... They've got to cope with a child being disfigured and injured and maimed plus their partner who doesn't know what to believe. ... I mean if we don't know what to believe and the police have been involved, then the partner's bound to think, are they capable of doing that sort of thing to a child?. .. Oh, I don't know, it's not just the problems that you see, like the disfigurement ... it must affect their whole life. (20, p. 43–45)

The difference between this nurse's perception of Sasha's mother and the general ward view was remarkable. She was able to revise her initial perceptions of the mother, not by reading her notes but by 'specialling' Sasha, by working closely with her mother and by standing within her world of concerns. She was able to 'just speak' to her and thus to learn more of the meaning of this traumatic experience for the mother's 'whole life'. I feel that the nurse has understood this well, and perhaps for this reason uses the burning metaphor of 'being engulfed' to describe how this mother felt. She also showed both sympathy and empathy for the mother as she has came to understand the many strains that bore upon her in relation to her daughter's future, her other children, her marriage and the possibility of some police investigation of the incident.

This finding of nurses' revising their perceptions of parents who had been initially judged and labelled as bad mothers was revealed in another nurse's account. The mother in this account had become what the nurse called 'the black sheep of the family' in relation to the other parents in the ward. Initially this nurse had shared the perceptions of other staff, that for example she should not have left the ward at night to join in local darts games:

She was going out in the evening (. . .) that was definitely frowned upon. I mean I'll be honest and say that I frowned upon it as well. (24, p. 27)

The nurse was also aware of other reasons behind the staff's negative perceptions:

There was a lot of nasty things said, you know, 'She wasn't here again today', you know ... and 'I don't know why we even bother giving her a key, we should take the room from her', and, you know, there was a lot of nasty things said. . . . I think it was her lifestyle, I think it was the number of men friends that she had as well that was frowned upon. . . . I think we all thought, If you've got x number of friends coming to see you, what is Ben's life going to be like at home? (24, p. 28–29)

The nurse described similar changes in her perceptions of this mother which developed as she got to know her and 'made an effort with her'. The nurse explained this.

Nurse: I didn't have as many problems with her as the rest of the staff did.
PD: Why would that be?
Nurse: I think it's 'cos I always made an effort with her and I always phoned her to come down and see to Ben and . . . I always made a point of going and speaking to her when she came into the ward (. . .) but I thought, it's a hard life being here all week, every day of the week, for the number of weeks that she was here, there isn't a life for them in the Mother's Unit and I think that the mothers judge each other up in the unit . . . and I think the other thing is that there's a bit of a clique between mothers that she never really fitted in . . . She had a few friends when Ben was first admitted and she kept in touch with them and that was who she used to go out with. . . . She never really made any friends after they left and I think she was really lonely up there. (24, p. 27–28)

A case conference was another occasion which afforded the nurse an insight into this mother's experience of hospitalization. I spoke to her in the ward after the conference and she explained that she

had never really understood what it was like for Ben's mum, being only 19 years old and being in this situation for over 14 weeks. (. . .) We [the nurses] asked an awful lot of her as a parent (. . .) she had a lot on her plate, not just with Ben but with the break-up of her marriage and with having other children at home.

She also spoke of how difficult it seemed to be for Ben's mum to talk to, confide in and discuss problems with the nurses (Fieldnote, 26/4/88).

It seemed that this case conference, for all its explicit and hidden agendas, had given the nurse a chance to really listen to and hear Ben's mother, not only as a live-in parent but also as a young woman of 19 whose life at the time was replete with problems. One result of the case conference was that Ben's mother and the nurse agreed that the nurse would take on the role of named person whom the mother could specifically approach to discuss any matters of concern. This was welcomed by the mother who felt that her best relationship was already with this nurse.

The nurse also welcomed this development as she believed that all parents, and especially those who had been living-in for a long time, should have such a 'primary nurse'. An unstated but equally important benefit was that this arrangement allowed the mother to circumvent another senior nurse with whom she had a very antagonistic relationship:

> And then the case conference, about the way she was treating Ben, there was a lot of grievances aired there . . . she had a lot of grievances about the staff in the ward and certainly we had a few, and once they were all out in the open and discussed . . . and then when I volunteered to be a go-between between her and [the other senior nurse] . . . I think things improved then. (24, p. 24–25)

3.4 CONCLUDING COMMENTS

The meaning of being a parent cannot be adequately captured in terms which are primarily instrumental or functional. While parents do indeed do things with their child, these are merely part of a wider kaleidoscope of intimacy and connection between the parent, child, family and society. I argue that being a parent is best understood ontologically and that the hospitalization of your child throws the moral dimension of being a parent into the sharpest relief. Parents are the child's protector and sustainer of life and their sense of moral adequacy as 'good parents' is frequently violated by the child's hospitalization.

Guilt seemed an all-pervasive accompaniment of every parental action or feeling. It was the proverbial 'rock and a hard place'. Parents felt guilty if they made a fuss and became a nuisance but also felt guilty if they accepted the situation and failed to 'fight for' their child. They felt guilty if they asked too many questions, if they imagined that they were not being useful enough, if their child was not as ill as others, if they treated them 'too normally', and if they had to leave their child for any reason. While some nurses' caring practices helped parents move in from the moral margins, for others there was little absolution from the guilt that they felt. Parents' guilt would not let them forget that 'if only they had . . .'. Parents whose child had developed a serious illness berated themselves for being on holiday when the illness developed, for having 'something wrong' with themselves which might have contributed to the child's illness or disease . . . for allowing whatever had happened to the child to happen.

If the parent–child relationship is characterized by power, then hospitalization shatters this mutual understanding. The parents no longer had the power to command the child, in this case to get well while the child was similarly powerless to ask their parents to make them better. Nor could parents continue to be their child's primary carer. This was now undertaken by professionals and parents could find themselves morally marginalized when they reflected on how their care might be measured against that of hospital staff and be found wanting. The hospital, its staff, its routines, other parents, their child, themselves, all could help to further erode the parent's sense of being a good parent. It seemed that the prevailing ethos of the hospital was a reflection of a wider current societal control paradigm or technological understanding (Taylor, 1989; Benner, 1990a) of human beings, in this case both staff and parents. This is not a reference to 'technological' in the sense of an ICU and its equipment. Within a technological understanding of persons, the self becomes objectified and mechanized. People become mere instruments or resources to be used and as such their way of being shows up for us in significantly different ways. Dreyfus (1991, p. 338) explained this well when he noted that 'we moderns encounter objects to be controlled and organized by subjects in order to satisfy their desires. Or, most recently as we enter the final stage of technology, we experience everything including ourselves as resources to be enhanced, transformed, and ordered simply for the sake of greater and greater efficiency.'

Parents seemed to sense this technological imperative soon after their admission when they were concerned to repay the privilege of being allowed to stay in by being seen to be functionally useful, both for their child and for the nurses. Such usefulness was, however, a poor substitute for a relationship with nurses which acknowledged human concerns, relatedness, connection and genuine involvement.

Nurses seemed to have a clear concept of the good live-in parent which reflected this technological understanding. The good resident parent was one who was there when required either by the child or staff, one who helped out when nurses were particularly busy but who was also able to avoid being over-involved either physically or emotionally. Their socially valued parental devotion (Brossat and Pinell, 1990) was never in doubt.

Parents were allowed to fall short in these areas but this tended to be only on occasions which were defined as legitimate by the nurses. For example, a nurse might have decided that a mother looked very tired and should go for a cup of coffee or that perhaps she had been living-in for too long and should go out for an evening with another parent or home for the weekend. Similarly parents might have been actively encouraged by a nurse to cry, to 'just let it all out' or to be angry, to 'get it all off their chest'. Under these circumstances and with nursing permission, parents could express feelings or behave in ways that might otherwise have earned them nurses' disapproval. It also seemed that parents were 'rationed' as to how often they might properly respond in such situations.

For many nurses, parents' suffering 'was a problem of management, not a crisis of spirit' (Frank, 1991, p. 131). A parent might have been forgiven and understood for having shouted at a nurse during a period of particular stress, or for asking a great many questions regarding their child's care, or for breaking down and crying when told some bad news, but it seemed that parents would not be allowed to exhibit such responses repeatedly without nurses' perceptions of them becoming more negative.

I argue that the moral dimension of being a live-in parent was not merely a private or idiosyncratic concern for parents. Nurses and parents together helped to create and shape parents' moral identities within the ward. This could be done in the most brutal and blatant of ways, for example by the nurse who made sure that her critical comments about a 'negligent' mother were loud enough to be heard by others. Moral disapproval was also expressed by the most fleeting of looks or facial expression, or by the most seemingly innocent but barbed remark. I have also shown that nurses assigned parents moral identities on the basis of performance criteria and that this was a perception shared largely by parents. However, live-in parents were often in the worst possible position to perform according to anyone's criteria. Parents were dwelling in their guilt, anguish, dread, and fear, trying somehow to manage these feelings in order to help comfort their child while simultaneously being a parent for the rest of their family. By contrast, many nurses stood outside parents' most primordial emotions and feelings and from this detached and professional vantage point, they were able to conceive of criteria that the 'good' or 'successful' parent should satisfy.

Parental involvement and participation

4

4.1 INTRODUCTION

Previous chapters have touched upon the importance of parent participation. This chapter suggests that parent participation, both in theory and in practice, is a more problematic and complex phenomenon than has previously been acknowledged.

I concentrate initially on the parents' and nurses' respective expectations and understandings of what parent participation would and did entail, exploring similarities and discordancies. I then extend this analysis in a discussion of the creation, control, and determination of parent participation. I argue that the interpretation of participants' accounts suggested that parent participation was more a set of unexpressed expectations than any form of mutual agreement between parents and nurses.

Parent participation, as a concept and as a professional tenet, begs the question of participation in what? Here, the parents' accounts of how they spent their days in the ward and how they perceived the nature of their participation were illuminating. I suggest that parental involvement, particularly in the early part of the child's stay, was limited to what I have called previously 'basic mothering work'.

Nurses often assumed that parents could carry out these familiar tasks equally well within the different context of the ward. However, I suggest that nurses' and parents' understandings and expectations of parental participation changed during the duration of the parents' stay in hospital in ways that calls this assumption into question.

The demarcation of care into basic mothering work and the more technical work of nursing or medical procedures was more clearly delineated in the earlier part of a parent's stay, becoming less pronounced over the length of the child's hospitalization. The strategies used by parents and nurses to bring about participation and its development are also discussed.

4.2 PARENTS' EXPERIENCES OF PARTICIPATION

I use two terms in this chapter 'participation' and 'involvement' as I suggest that, for the research participants, there was a subtle but nonetheless important distinction between them. I take participation to refer to the more functional involvement of parents in their child's care, for example in helping carry out their everyday care. For the parents, I suggest that involvement had a more holistic connotation, implying a deeper sense of being an integral and essential part of their child's hospital experience. It is parental involvement in this deeper sense that is discussed here. This section describes how parent participation was created, controlled and experienced by both parents and nurses.

While the parents had a general desire to help to care for their child during their stay, they may have lacked sufficient or specific knowledge of the child's condition to allow them to do this confidently. Being a live-in parent was not a static 'role', however. Changes in the child's condition, the length of the parent's stay and parent's relationships with ward staff all influenced the nature of parents' participation. Just as parents' moral status within the ward could change, as was shown in Chapter 3, so parents' participation was not a fixed but a dynamic state. During the period of fieldwork I met many parents whose levels and kinds of participation were different. Some were very happy to carry out only their child's basic mothering care and leave the more technical care to nurses while others had learned some technical skills, such as nasogastric feeding, in order that they could do this with their child.

There were also a small group of parents who had attained the status of what I will call 'expert parents', whose autonomy and expertise regarding their child's care marked them out as being quite unique. This concept of the expert parent has important implications for the more general discussion of parental participation, and will be discussed at the end of this chapter.

For the majority of parents, becoming increasingly involved in their child's care was an uncertain process. During the interviews and discussions with parents I asked them to tell me about how they spent their day, which would usually elicit some information as to how the parents participated, if at all, in their child's care. I might also ask how it came about that they began to do the particular things that they did for their child.

4.2.1 Determining participation: parents' understandings

The parents who chose to live-in with their child in hospital seemed to have no clear idea as to what the nature or extent of their participation in their child's care might be. Some parents' ideas prior to living-in reflected fairly outmoded concepts of paediatric care. For example some expressed pleasant surprise at being 'allowed' to do so much for their child. As one mother noted:

> I was surprised . . . this is the first time I've been in hospital and I was surprised that they let the mothers do so much to tell you the truth . . .

just because I didn't know what to expect, I mean, I thought a mother came to hospital and sat with her child all day and done nothing for her child, that they [the nurses] did everything . . . and I was quite pleasantly surprised to see that they allow you to do so much for them. (Mother 4, 27, p. 25)

Parent participation did not appear to be an openly negotiated arrangement. Parents therefore had the task of steering an appropriate course through the uncertain and, as was often the case, uncharted area of participation in their child's care.

At no time did any parent mention that they had specifically asked to participate in a particular aspect of their child's care and been disallowed from doing so. However, there were occasions when parents expressed criticisms concerning institutional barriers to their participation. Recall the previous discussion of the ward kitchens.

When I asked parents how they came to do the things that they did for their child in hospital, they usually replied that this was an automatic or instinctive reaction. They tried to carry on normally by providing the same care that they had been providing at home prior to their admission. As these parents explained:

My wife just took it upon herself (. . .) typical mother, like, she just got up and done it, like, with no asking. (12, p. 24)

Just naturally (. . .) natural instinct. (Mother 2 and Father 3, 25, p. 7)

I just did it automatically, he was my son, it was my responsibility. (6, p. 30)

These replies might seem to indicate that for parents there was a seamless continuity between their child-care practices at home and in the hospital. However, this was often not the case and parents often found the process of participating in their child's care to be fraught with tensions. They were often uncertain and confused as to what exactly they were allowed and expected to do. Consequently, parents regularly remarked that they had learned the limits of their participation by the often chastening experience of trial and error. For example, they might have been chastized for using the ward kitchen.

For the majority of the parents, parent participation was an unspoken agreement. These parents' comments were representative:

You're not told, basically, and they don't ask you what you would like. . . . If they would say, 'Do you want to feed your child every meal yourself?' 'Do you want to do this and that?' I mean, if you weren't here they would have to. (26, p. 38)

No, no, no, that [the mother's level of participation] was never discussed, never discussed, I just did everything.(. . .) No, it was never mentioned, Philip, I just took it as being the way. (14, p. 14–15)

I don't think anything was said like that, I think it's just expected that if a parent's there they'll do things. (. . .) It's as if you're here and you're going to have to do it all. (2, p. 43)

Parents would also watch what other resident parents did for their child and take their cues from them. The nature of their participation was also determined by the severity of the child's illness or injury. Generally, the more seriously ill the child was, the less directly the parents would participate, even in basic mothering work. One mother's comments illustrated this clearly in relation to her baby son who was in an intensive care unit:

There was nothing we could do, he was on a ventilator, he was so sick . . . he didn't need us at all, it's just that we were there 'cos we thought that every breath could be his last one . . . and we felt that we had to be with him. It's different now [at this time the baby was in a close observation area within the main ward], I can do things for him, I can change his nappy and I can give him his feeds down his NG tube, but that's still not really **doing** anything. (17, p. 5–6)

This mother's account was also illustrative of the ways in which the ethos of the ward tended to elevate the importance of the technical task or the physical procedure. Within such an ethos, parents' presencing with their child, their bearing witness beside him when his hold on life was at its most fragile was less valued and under-recognized. Their presence seemed synonymous with a useless passivity, a 'doing nothing' for their baby who 'didn't need' them.

Parents participated more when they were asked informally and unthreateningly by nurses as to whether they might like to help with a particular aspect of their child's care. This encouragement also extended to the performance of more technical tasks such as the giving of nasogastric feeds, although parents tended to be taught more formally how to carry out these procedures, rather than gently encouraged. Two mothers described this strategy:

The nurse just said one day, 'I'm going to wash Claire, do you want to help?' and I said, 'That's fine, am I allowed to?', and she said, 'Well, we quite encourage the mums to take part and do things with their kids.' (Mother 2, 27, p. 20–21)

At first they always cleaned her and then they sort of said, 'Do you want to do it?' and I sort of said, 'It doesn't bother me,' and they said, 'We're just sort of cleaning her,' so I sort of took over. (10, p. 33)

The ways in which nurses broached the subject of the parents' participating were important to parents. They were appreciative of nurses who allowed them to make their own choices as to whether and to what degree they wished to participate. It was particularly important in this respect that the parents were allowed to decide their own level of participation without feeling that were being pressurized. In this way they were able to vary their participation depending upon how they were feeling at any given time. These parents' accounts illustrated this point:

> **Mother:** There are more things that I can do and there are more things that I'm encouraged to do, which I like (. . .) so they're maybe just little things but I can do more now which makes me feel a bit more necessary.
> **PD:** Were you actually encouraged to do these things, did someone come up and say. . . ?
> **Mother:** Well, no – well, yes . . . encouraged . . . they would say, 'You can do this if you want to.'
> **PD:** Uhuh
> **Mother:** You know, they didn't say, 'Right, change his nappy,' and if at any time I don't want to, I can just say, 'No, I don't want to.' (17, p. 24–25) They'll not say, 'Right you'll do it!' . . . they'll say, 'Do you want to finish off or do you want me to carry on?' and I'll say aye. . . . It's a wee bit of give and take. (15, p. 57–58)

It would have been almost unthinkable for parents to have taken it upon themselves to carry out aspects of their child's care that might have been thought the prerogative of nurses. This was not only the more traditionally nursing tasks such as changing dressings and recording observations. Live-in parents quickly realized that what would previously have been considered basic mothering tasks, such as feeding, changing and bathing the child, now required nurses' permission if they were to be done by parents.

One way for parents to legitimize their participation was for them to portray their involvement, not as interference in the working of the ward but as being of positive help to nurses. As these mothers noted:

> I mean, you know that you're helping them, because one nurse maybe gets three bairns but all she has to do with my one is take her temperature and pulse and she can devote all her time to the other two, 'cos I'm in here the whole day, virtually seven o'clock in the morning till eight at night and on call if they want me. (12, p. 21)

> I dare say it takes a strain away from them as well towards that child (. . .) and they can spend more time with another child. (14, p. 14–15)

It seemed important for parents to find a balance in the level of their participation in their child's care. If this balance was upset then they might feel that they were being expected to carry out too much of the child's care without adequate support. One mother described her feelings of being virtually her child's sole carer while in hospital:

> Well, I think I **have** been his carer (laughs), I've been the one that's done it really (. . .) but I still think that there should be a back-up from the nursing staff (. . .) sometimes I wish that someone would come and give him a bath and, you know, just get him changed. (2, p. 40–41)

As was shown in Chapter 2, the need to participate to some degree was explained by some parents as being one of the prime justifications for their deciding to live-in, as this mother explained:

> When you come in, you change them and things, nurses will say, 'Do you want a hand?' and you'll say, 'No, I can manage on my own', because if you **didn't** do that, you wouldn't be helping at all, if they said to you, 'We'll change her and change her nappy and wash her and things, leave that all to us' . . . all you would do all day would be sit there. (4, p. 6–7)

As the following nurses' accounts suggested, the control and determination of the extent and level of parent participation seemed to lie principally with nursing staff. However, parents did carry out some of their child's care on their own initiative, for example one mother told how she had decided to wash her child without seeking permission:

> Jill was in here for about three days before I realized that nobody had washed her, I mean I'd washed her face when she'd been sick but nobody had come and washed her, and as soon as I had filled up the basin one of the nurses came up and helped, but I made the decision. (Mother 4, 27, p. 22–23)

Another mother took this a stage further by initiating her own form of treatment for her comatose son, believing that in the absence of any other explicit treatment plan, she was obliged to do her best to devise something:

> Nobody has come up to me and said, 'Look, we think this might be a good idea, if you talk about this or do this with John,' there's nobody come over and suggested anything like that. (. . .) I've taken it upon my own back to take him out of his chair and walk him a couple of steps or put him in his bed for a little while. (4, p. 4–5)

Taking such participatory initiatives was not an easy option as it could render the parent open to suggestions that they were overstepping the mark and encroaching into areas that were proper concerns of nursing and medical staff. One of the ways in which parents avoided creating such a situation was by ensuring that nurses were consulted and informed about any care that the parents wished to give their child. One mother, who was herself a nurse, but not a paediatric nurse, explained how she negotiated her participation by effectively denying her ability to carry out some of her child's technical care. This ensured that even if she had taken her child's temperature, the nurses would follow this up by doing it 'properly' and entering the official result in the child's chart:

> I have to be really careful and not breach their territory, because I'm quite capable of taking his temperature and his pulse. The first night I came in, the doctor, he had said, 'You could just fill in his chart for me,' and I thought, I don't have a pen and I was glad I didn't have a pen 'cos you don't

know how people are going to react in those situations (. . .) and after that I made sure I didn't have a pen because I didn't want to step over that line because in here I don't think they would like it one bit if I did. . . . I take his temp, but the nurses take it after me, I don't mind, I just say, 'Oh, I took his temp', but that's all. I don't interfere with the charts, no, I just don't. (. . .) I think my reason for that is the attitude of the [ward] hierarchy, shall we put it. The attitude to me is, 'Well, she's a nurse and just watch her.' (. . .) I just really feel uncomfortable (. . .) it's, 'She's a bit of a know-all, she thinks she knows a bit about everything . . . just step over that line a bit. . . . (6, p. 22–23)

Most parents were aware that they were performing a delicate social balancing act and thought it prudent to try to keep on the good side of nurses. Having described how the phenomenon of parent participation came about, I now explore, from the parents' perspective, what such participation actually entailed.

4.2.2 Parents and play: 'worse than working'

The importance of play for hospitalized children has been repeatedly emphasized in recent years (Jolly, 1981; Betz and Poster, 1984; Department of Health, 1991). Paediatric nurses have been encouraged to attend to the play and recreational needs of children as well as to their more physical needs. The introduction of play leaders in paediatric hospitals (Hall, 1977) has been another attempt to ensure that children's play needs are not neglected.

The literature on play has, however, tended to ignore or take for granted the active part that live-in parents play in keeping their child amused and occupied during their stay. Previous studies of play have also tended to characterize play solely as a diversionary activity for the child and have ignored the importance of the meanings which play had for parents. I suggest that these meanings were tightly bound to parents' understandings of their child's condition and prognosis and to their own lived experience of being resident parents. In this section I therefore describe not only parents' involvement in play but, equally importantly, the ways in which parents' understandings of play could be altered by the nature of their child's condition.

Most parents will attest to the fact that keeping a young child amused, occupied or entertained for a sustained length of time is not an easy task. For live-in parents this was made much more difficult by virtue of the child's illness, possibly restricted mobility and the physical restrictions of an unfamiliar environment. It was difficult for some parents to play with their child for long periods of time as this pattern of interaction was so different from that which they usually experienced at home.

While a child will certainly interrupt their mother for drinks, for help with toys and for comfort if they have an accident, this pattern of play interaction is not so concentrated as that described by live-in parents. One mother described the intensity of this contact when her child had been admitted for one of his earlier operations:

> **PD:** Apart from the sort of physical things, the sort of washing and changing etcetera . . . what other kinds of things do you find yourself doing for Steven?
> **Mother:** Playing games . . . now, a lot of the time he just plays himself, like, and with the other kids, but when he was younger [this refers to an earlier hospital admission] it [playing with and amusing the child] was like from the minute you were in till the minute you were out. (13, p. 35)

Another mother described a similar intensity of play involvement with her child:

> **PD:** How did you find that you spent your day while you were here?
> **Mother:** By her bedside, as I say, half six in the morning till she went and slept at night, with the odd break in between, playing games with her. (14, p. 12–13)

This mother's daughter had received a skin graft and consequently had to lie in a fairly uncomfortable position on her tummy that considerably restricted her mobility and scope for independent play activity. This mother's account hinted that such playing and amusing were often extremely hard work for parents, who were usually more accustomed to their children playing on their own or with friends.

The parents of the comatose children who had sustained serious head injuries explained that there was no demarcation between verbal stimulation and play. Most of their efforts to amuse or play with their child centred on trying to elicit any kind of response that could be favourably interpreted. Their major difficulty was in speaking to and stimulating their child, who before the accident had been active and talkative and who was now almost entirely unresponsive.

> **PD:** What about the other things . . . you mentioned stimulating, talking . . . how do those things compare?
> **Mother:** Worse. That is worse than working. The hardest thing in there is sitting talking to Kim . . . because you know looking at her that she's lying sleeping, and it makes you tired, you really feel exhausted, you know I just talk to her as much as I can and then I put her tapes on . . . I think, if she's lying there and she's listening to something it'll make her feel that there's no nobody sitting at all with her.
> **Father:** It makes you feel as if you're helping her, even if it's just a tape you're playing her.
> **Mother:** What do you say next? You've spoke about **every possible thing** you could say to her . . . what do you do next? (5, p. 34–35)

The mother of another child with a head injury expressed similar feelings in relation to stimulating her son:

> I should be here because nobody else has got the time to sit with John, literally sit, not change or feed or anything like that . . . sit and talk, about

anything at all. I've repeated so many things now so many times he's probably fed up with me (laughs) . . . but you try to think of what happened the day before and then you talk about that and you sort of get stuck so you go back to things that you know you've said before but that he might not have taken in at the time. (4, p. 6)

The importance of the meaning of play within the context of the child's illness was memorably demonstrated during my interview with this mother. She was almost in tears, partly sadness and partly anger, as she told me how she had come into the ward one day to find her son, who was approximately 10 years old, holding, and in her view being expected to play with, a pillow. 'Can you believe that, a pillow!' She repeated this phrase several times as if she could scarcely comprehend the implications of what she had seen.

For this mother, play was not merely a diversion to amuse or entertain her child, it also had a normalizing function. This mother was adamant that her son should not have been given toys like rattles or activity centres because, as she said, 'he's not a baby'. Despite the fact that he was only just beginning to regain rudimentary purposive motor functions, his mother refused to see this as a second babyhood and insisted on age-appropriate toys for her son. Play for her was clearly not only a part of her child's therapy but an important part of the construction or more properly, the reconstruction of her child's identity.

For another parent whose baby was developmentally delayed, her sense of involvement in his care revolved around play and stimulation that could not, or may not have been given by nurses. She had a clear perception that playing with and amusing her child was not merely an activity to pass the time or to stave off boredom but that it was an important stimulus for her child's developmental progress.

> **Mother:** I feel quite involved. I can only say I'm glad I'm here, 100% glad.
> **PD:** Why?
> **Mother:** Because I know he's getting total attention, which is impossible for the nurses to give him. He doesn't need a great deal of attention, Alan will happily lie there, but when he just lies there he goes backwards, so he's got to have something on the go, somebody speaking, somebody rattling something in front of him . . . anything at all . . . .
> **PD:** So if you weren't here what would happen?
> **Mother:** He'd lie there, he'd get the mobile turned on, the dummy put in his mouth and that would be it. (6, p. 4–5)

Play was also used by parents as a diversionary tactic to distract their child and to hopefully minimize the distress of painful or frightening procedures. Here, a parent described how she used play to lessen her daughter's fear of being anaesthetized:

> When we got into the anaesthetic room she just screamed and burst into tears and there was no way . . . . We tried a little game, you know, blow up

the bag on the thing, look it's a big balloon, try and blow it up for Mummy, but no. . . . (10, p. 62)

Another mother explained how she perceived playing and amusing her child as being similarly an attempt to divert her daughter's thoughts from the potentially distressing aspects of her treatment.

My main worry at that time was Alice. . . . I'd have to keep her mind occupied, I'd have to keep her mind busy to keep her mind off what was wrong with her, and I worried about that. (14, p. 5)

Parents also used play interactions as a way of monitoring changes in their child's condition. For example one mother detected an improvement in her child when her daughter became less dependent upon her constant attention and began to show an interest in playing with some of the other children on the ward.

The first week or so she just wasn't interested in who was going past [the cubicle], she just wanted Mummy and she just wanted someone to sit and read to her, play with her, a few games, but towards the end of the time she would watch people going past, and sort of, if one of the little ones came up to the glass and waved to her, she would wave frantically and the girl round the corner was called Jill and if she saw her it would be 'Look, Mummy, look, there's Jill!' . . . and she was obviously starting to feel better and want more contact. (10, p. 18–19)

Parents' stay in hospital was temporary and they anticipated the difficulties that might arise when they returned home with their child. A common parental concern here was that the child had become accustomed to having the virtually constant and compliant attention of their mother for several days or even weeks. The previous mother described how she tried to gradually withdraw her attention as the child's condition improved. In this way she hoped that the child would become less dependent upon her for play.

I tried not to play with her constantly, so that, if she can amuse herself a bit, let her do it, 'cos I don't want her, sort of, have her feeling that she was going to have me constantly there. (. . .) If she was playing with something I would just sit and read or sit and knit. I would sort of push the chair back so that I wasn't totally with her, playing with her, so that she would play on her own for a bit. (10, p. 17, 20–21)

If the phrase parent participation begs the question, participation in what? then the parents' accounts of their experiences and understandings of play provided a partial answer.

Parents did not view play merely as something to keep their child occupied for the duration of their day. They saw it as being integral to many other aspects of the child's condition, treatment and recovery. In keeping with a central tenet of this study, play had unique, context-specific meanings for parents that could easily be overlooked if it were seen as a purely functional or instrumental part of parent participation.

4.2.3 Basic mothering: doing 'the natural mother things'

When asked to describe the kinds of things that they did for their child, as opposed to the things that nurses did, parents would usually describe basic mothering. Parents depicted basic mothering work as a continuation of their normal lives out-with the hospital.

> **PD:** What would you say has been your main function while you've been here?
> **Mother:** Just his mum. Looking after him as I would at home. (2, p. 32)
> **PD:** How did you know to do the things that you do for your child . . . did someone say?
> **Mother 3:** It's an automatic reaction.
> **Mother 4**: You would do it for them in your house, so you go and do it here. (28, p. 14)

The child's condition was an important influence here, for if the child was not viewed as being seriously ill, then it seemed easier for parents to carry on normally with the basic mothering aspects of their child's care. For other parents, however, the nature of their child's illness or injury had an impact upon their ability to simply carry on as if they were at home, as this mother made clear in her account:

> I just automatically did it [her daughter's physical care]. . . . I was **very**, **very** wary of . . . I didn't mind feeding her at the top end or washing her down to the waist or anything like that, but anything near the burn area I was very wary about (. . .) her bottom was exposed you know and I was very sort of wary, if she moved her bowels or anything. At first they always cleaned her and then they sort of said, 'Do you want to do it?' and I sort of said, 'It doesn't bother me [I don't care one way or the other],' and they said, 'We're just sort of cleaning her,' so I sort of took over . . . but I wouldn't have anything to do with . . . not because I didn't want to, but because I didn't want the sort of risks of doing more damage, and I was very wary of doing anything with the bottom half. (10, p. 32–33)

Carrying on as normal with the child's basic mothering care was also made diffi-cult by the strange surroundings and routines of the ward. Where parents had not been given sufficient information regarding the routine and layout of the ward, then even the simplest of tasks, such as giving their child a wash or bath were made difficult, as this mother explained:

> There's questions like going for a bath. . . . the first day I waited thinking that a nurse would come (. . .) not necessarily to help me but to show me

where I could find a towel, show me, you know . . . if I had stuff to put in the bath or what have you, but because I was there as a parent I was left to get on with it. (26, Mother 1, p. 27–28)

The desire to participate by carrying out basic mothering tasks created a sense of ambivalence for parents. While they were willing to help in this way and believed that this was an important part of their role, I have previously described how at times they felt undervalued and exploited.

Basic mothering work was described by parents as being one of the most important ways in which they participated in their child's care. However, as I have previously argued, parent participation was not static but dynamic. Parents become involved not only in the child's basic everyday care but in what were regarded, at least initially, as the more technical aspects of the child's care. That some activities and tasks were viewed as being more technical and therefore within the domain of nurses and doctors was a perception not only of parents, but as I shall later show, also of some nurses. The following section discusses the nature of parent participation in relation to these technical tasks.

4.2.4 Technical tasks: 'the medical things'

Few parents described themselves as playing a particularly active part in the more technical aspects of their child's care and most conceived of such work as being outwith both their remit and expertise. Two mothers in one of the group interviews expressed some surprise when I asked whether there was a difference between the kind of things that nurses did for their child and the things that they did as parents. They brought out clearly that there were lines of demarcation:

Mother 3: I do the natural mother things, they do the medical things that you are not experienced to.
Mother 4: Well, that's their job, you wouldn't think of doing things like that.(. . .) There's definitely a difference between what you'll do and what you'll not do, you don't interfere in that side of it. (28, p. 22–23)

Parents also felt that there was a different and essentially lesser value attached to their child-care practices compared with the work of nursing and medical staff. One mother expressed this stark differential when she explained that she did

the, sort of, non-essential things like changing nappies. . . . I mean, they're keeping him alive, basically, and I'm doing all the little fiddly bits to keep him mildly comfortable and talking to him and trying to comfort him, which isn't easy 'cos he's so . . . but they keep doing all the important things, keeping him alive. (Mother 17, p. 33–34)

One way in which parents closed this perceived gap between the nature of their work and nurses' 'important' work was to gradually become more conversant with technical tasks.

Examples of this were apparent in the accounts of parents of children who had spent some days or even weeks in an intensive care unit. These parents often learned the language of the unit and became more conversant with its technology. I suggest here that this may have been done in order to better understand the nature of what was happening to their child in this new and strange world. I also suggest that parents learned the language and ways of the ICU in order to become more valued observers of their child's condition from the perspective of the ICU staff. A mother gave this account of what happened when her baby 'went off' or 'took a wobbly' as she described it:

> His saturation drops and he starts to struggle for breath . . . it's a build up of secretions, a clot that has to be removed by a combination of physiotherapy, suction and nebulizer to break it up . . . and it happens within five minutes, because the last one he threw in the ward that got him back into ICU . . . his saturation had been 100 . . . and his colour had been acceptable and all his observations had been fine. Five minutes later his saturations were dropping like a stone and he was grey and needed urgent help. (Mother 17, p. 18)

This is an account that could equally have come from a nurse giving a change of shift report and is in marked contrast to the mother's initially more informal description of the event that the baby was 'taking a wobbly'. The previously mentioned concept of a knowledge value differential seems pertinent again here. If a parent wished to become a valued participant in a highly specialist area such as an ICU, which is linguistically as well as technically alien to parents, it was a valuable strategy to try to adapt to this new situation by learning its discourse. In this way parents could develop a better understanding of some of the unfamiliar jargon and procedures which they would encounter. They also equipped themselves with a vocabulary and level of technical understanding that might ensure that their comments and observations were treated with more respect by staff.

Parents who undertook more technical tasks were those whose children were expected to be in hospital for longer periods. These were, for example, children admitted following a severe scald or head injury, or those who had a chronic illness which might necessitate future hospital admissions, or where the child might have to have some form of treatment carried out at home by the parents. For the parents of a comatose child recovering from a head injury, it was important for themselves as well as for their child that they be allowed to do some of the more technical tasks in order that they could feel more fully involved in her care. As her father explained:

> We wanted to do jobs instead of just sitting there. (. . .) Once we realized that it was going to be a long, long thing we felt that we'd be better asking the nurses what we could do, what they could show us what to do, so that we felt as if we were helping Kim, and through her we were helping ourselves as well, you know. (Father 10, p. 3)

Technical work seemed to be largely controlled by medical and nursing staff. Parents who wished to undertake these kinds of tasks would be assessed by nurses as to whether they would be capable of performing the tasks safely and competently (Webb *et al.*,1985). The initial approach to undertake these tasks may have come from nurses who felt that it was time the parents learned how to carry out this procedure or from the parents themselves who were keen to perform the task.

Parents described how carrying out these tasks made them feel that they were participating more valuably in the care of their child while, again, feeling that they were 'helping out' the nurses. A father emphasized both of the above points when he described his feelings as he was offered the chance to feed his daughter:

> I'm really happy, like, with what happened today. . . . I walked in and just as I walked in the wee nurse had brought her feed up, so that was me delighted 'cos I knew that I'd be able to feed her so it was a case of walking up to the nurse and saying, 'I'll do that' . . . 'Oh, that's fine, Mr White, that lets me get on' [the nurse replied], so I felt delighted then, whereas if I come in and she's had her feed she isn't due another one for four hours and I've got to get away . . . when I go out of here, if I've not done nothing [anything], you feel . . . really down because you've not actually done nothing. (5, p. 33–34)

Nurses were also happy to allow parents to take over nursing tasks where it was thought that the child was liable to become particularly troublesome or distressed. One mother, who was also a general practitioner and therefore deemed competent to carry out the task, was allowed to take her son's temperature:

> I mean, Peter's getting really stroppy with everyone that's coming up to him, so if he doesn't want his temperature taken, I mean the nurses are quite happy for me to stick the thermometer under his arm, just little things like that, just to make him feel a little bit more at ease. (27, Mother 1, p. 23)

As with basic mothering, parents' participation in more technical aspects of their child's care was variable and dependent upon several factors. Important here were the nature and severity of the child's illness, the parent's keenness to become involved in such tasks and the willingness of nurses to facilitate this sharing. From the parents' perspective it seemed that there was a clear demarcation between nurses' work and parents' work. It was also clear that parents required to exercise tact and care if they were to successfully negotiate to undertake some of their child's technical care. A particular question that arose from this section was whether parents and nurses had similar or conflicting understandings of this demarcation. I examine this question later in the chapter.

While parents often described the more distinctly active aspects of participation, such as basic mothering work, there was also an important element of participation that involved the parent's 'being there' for their child in a more existential sense. This was an aspect of parents' experiences of living-in that the professional literature on parent participation has largely ignored, underplayed or characterized as being synonymous with boredom and inactivity (Meadow, 1969; 1974).

In the following section I counter this view and show that keeping vigil and being there with their child were, for parents, both symbolically and functionally important aspect of participation.

4.2.5 Keeping vigil

Parents who were carrying out their child's physical care or who were actively helping nurses with technical procedures were participating in highly visible ways. There were occasions however, when parents felt themselves to be intensely involved with their child, yet may have seemed to be merely sitting beside the child's bed. The accounts of the parents in this study suggested that keeping vigil or being with the child was not simply a matter of the parents being in close physical proximity to the child's bed, but was rather a bearing witness that often involved the most intense emotions.

Parents were often being with or presencing themselves with their child in the existential sense (Reimen, 1982; Benner, 1984; Benner and Wrubel, 1989) where they were hyperattentive to their child, acutely sensitive to their needs, at times to the point where they seemed to exclude all other aspects of their environment. This was especially so when the child was seriously ill. One mother conveyed this well when she described a time when her baby's life was considered to be in real danger:

> **PD:** While you were there [in the ICU], what did you actually do?
> **Mother:** Nothing (laughs nervously), just sort of sat and watched him . . . cried a lot . . . wandered about . . . just in total turmoil . . . we couldn't do anything, we could just sit. . . . We just sat and either watched him or sat and just thought (. . .) never said a word really, just sat and watched him. . . . (17, p. 5, 8)

This powerful need to be with their child and to be there for them was expressed by several other parents. One father whose son had been badly scalded and who had been taken immediately from Casualty into the ward treatment room expressed the distress that he felt when he was unable to be with his son at a moment when he felt that his child most needed him:

> So we got to the hospital and they put us in a wee room at the side and the wean [child] was screaming and at this you were getting all tense and tense, **you want to go in, you want to go in**. (18, p. 3–4)

This father also expressed a typical desire to be there for his child during the 'tough times' when the child was most likely to be frightened, perhaps when undergoing a painful or distressing procedure.

For some parents, the desire to keep vigil with their child had a strong functional importance. They were very keen to work in some way with their child as well as to be available to respond to the child's other needs and wishes. One parent described an experience shared by many other parents when she described how the need to be beside her child was so strong that she could not detach herself enough, in any sense, to relax and enjoy a short coffee break.

> You think, 'Oh, I'll just go for a drink' and then when you're in there you're thinking to yourself, 'I shouldn't be sat here, I should be sat in there talking, or doing something.' (4, p. 13)

Another mother explained how she tried to go home for a short break and to be with her other children for a while but found this impossible:

> I can't cook, Philip, I can't do it. I try to force myself . . . but if I'm in the house for any length of time I start breaking down about Kim and I've got to come right back in again. (5, p. 31)

An important feature of keeping vigil was the length of time that parents spent in often concentrated attention at their child's bedside. A father whose daughter was comatose spoke of sitting 'for maybe four . . . five hours or whatever' when he visited the hospital. His wife also described how, when her daughter had developed a serious infection, she had 'sat with her for 12 hours one day'. She also brought out clearly in her account the unique meaning that the experience of keeping vigil had for her sense of being a parent:

> I've seen some mammies coming in with their babies and just walking out and leaving them crying . . . maybe they've got important things in the house to do but I couldn't do that. I've got to sit with her, right up to 11 o'clock at night to make sure she's going to sleep, then I can go to sleep, but I can't come away till she's settled. But I wouldn't do that in the house, I would just say 'Get to bed!' and that would be it, whereas in here. . . . (5, p. 50–51)

Parents also spoke of when they simply had to be with their child at particularly significant moments, times that could not be formalized within a framework of 'functional reasons'. For one mother this was on the anniversary of her father's death:

> I'm sitting up in the Mothers' Unit and I'm bored and I've seen me going in to sit beside him at one or two in the morning, just thinking about what's happened . . . likes of on Saturday, there, I went in at one o'clock in the morning, and I sat with him till four o'clock, just sat and bubbled [snivelled] and cried 'cos it was five years ago on Saturday that my dad died . . . and it was the first year that I'd missed going to the crematorium 'cos I was through here with Ben. (. . .) I just sat and, the way he was lying, I just held his hand . . . and I just sat there and bubbled and cried, I couldn't help myself. (15, p. 63–64)

This mother needed to be with her son at this particularly significant time in her life. Through this moment of vigil with her child she experienced a sense of connectedness that seemed to help her to cope with a particularly traumatic time. Nurses often expressed the hope, that parents would 'come to terms with' their child's illness or death. It is possible that this mother had found the act of keeping vigil and being with her son at this quiet and relatively private time to be a help as she tried to understand and 'come to terms' with the circumstances surrounding his accident and injuries. It also seemed that being with her child had been a source of comfort to her as she remembered her father and his death.

I argue here that keeping vigil was not the passive, uninvolved, non-activity that some previous studies have suggested (Meadow, 1969). Keeping vigil served several purposes for parents although its meaning cannot be adequately captured in purely instrumental terms. It was a way of dwelling attentively and receptively with their child. It also helped the parents themselves to feel useful. By keeping vigil with their child parents felt that they were not only doing the right thing in the moral sense but the only thing that they could do. They were being of real help to their child at what were among the most traumatic moments of both of their lives.

4.2.6 Breaks and meals: 'no rest for the wicked'

Recognition of the taxing nature of being a live-in parent led me to ask parents how they managed coffee breaks and mealtimes. This is another aspect of living-in and participation that has been deemed unproblematic and has consequently been ignored in the research literature. The parents showed however, that this was both an important and often difficult aspect of living-in.

There were clearly limits as to how long parents could spend at their child's bedside without having to take at least a short break. Such breaks, however, were often of limited value to parents for there was little relaxation or 'charging of the batteries' done during these breaks. Instead, parents reported feeling guilty about having taken a break at all, or told how they would rush to gulp down a cup of coffee or smoke a quick cigarette before hurrying back to the bedside. Some parents spoke of how they found it 'too depressing' to sit in the parents' coffee lounge as the topic of conversation was invariably other children's illnesses and injuries.

Parents were usually unwilling to take a break from the ward unless their child was napping or unless a nurse or other parent was watching over them. Thus, as the following parents' comments show, the child effectively determined when and even if parents were allowed a meal or coffee break.

You have to go when the child will allow you to. (Mother 1, (26, p. 81)

We had to restrict them [breaks] till when Sally was asleep. (12, p. 18)

You just go when the bairn's settled. (Mother 2, p. 40)

This inability to take breaks and meals as necessary led some parents to describe the resultant ill-effects that this had on their general wellbeing. This also occurred at a time when parents needed to feel at their best in order to deal with the stresses of living-in with their child. Parents spoke of not eating properly, or not eating at all, of going 12 hours and more without eating or drinking or of resorting to unremitting junk food. Two mothers described a common reluctance to leave their child unattended or to even ask a nurse to watch their child while they went for a break:

> I just about **starved** to death the first couple of days . . . just . . . I mean, it was my own fault really, 'cos I wouldn't leave the wee one. There was always going to be something else happening and I thought . . . if he gets upset I'd better be there when it finishes'. (Mother 1, 27, p. 31)

> There was one day I couldn't get any of the visitors to look after the wee chap so I could go for something to eat and it was about six o'clock at night and nurse said, 'You look awful, are you OK?' and I said, 'No, actually I feel awful and I think I'm going to pass out,' and she said, 'Oh, you've just gone a funny colour,' and I said, 'What time is it?' and I said, 'It's OK, it's just because I haven't eaten all day' – because none of my family had come to take the child from me, and I didn't think to say to a nurse, 'Could you watch him till I go for something to eat?' (Mother 5, 26, p. 80–81)

Other mothers described how their normal nutritional habits had altered for the worse during their stay. This was often attributed to the restricted menus on offer in the hospital canteen and to the pressure that parents felt to get meals and breaks over with as quickly as possible in order to return to their child's bedside.

> Absolutely horrendous. I mean, I've put on loads of weight just because I've been eating loads of junk food. (. . .) I mean, I only cook chips once a week at home, twice at most . . . but since I've come in here all I've eaten is chips and fried stuff and yeeeech!, 'cos they don't do salads or anything in the canteen and it's absolutely . . . really awful. (10, p. 24)

These complaints may seem unreasonable. Surely parents could have gone else-where for meals, for example to one of the small cafés or take-aways that were within easy walking distance of the hospital? This however, ignores parents' powerful desire to remain as close to their child as possible. Parents might even-tually have felt able to leave the ward for a short while to visit a nearby tea-room or canteen within the hospital, but it was far more difficult for parents to bring themselves to leave the hospital building.

The parents' worst possible scenario was that something serious would happen to their child while they were out enjoying a break and could not be contacted. Even relatively minor problems caused parents to feel guilty at having left their child to take a break. One mother described how she felt when she learned that her son had vomited while she had been out of the hospital:

> You make yourself all (gestures anxiety) . . . you say, 'Was that because I went out for something to eat?' see, he just had a wee vomit this morning

and ate all day long. (. . .) I went out at quarter to nine for some quick fish and chips, and there, he had vomited all everywhere when I was out, and I thought, 'I wonder if he got himself into a state 'cos I had went out? (Mother 4, 28, p. 13)

Such flings caused some parents never to leave the hospital building and parent participation became an all-or-nothing phenomenon. To participate in your child's care and to be a good parent was to be with your child constantly.

During these breaks, parents' thoughts were invariably of their child and how they should be returning to the ward:

PD: See when you actually get away for your dinner or a cup of coffee, is that really a break?'
Mother: No, no because you're shovelling it down your throat to get back again.
Father: It's as quick as I can get out and as quick as I can get back again.
PD: Do you find that you can switch off for 10 minutes when you go for a cup of coffee?
Mother: No, I don't, no. (2, p. 47)

Breaks were therefore stolen moments from the essential task of being constantly with the child. As this mother explained:

I suppose it is important that I eat but . . . . . . you know, Sean comes first, you know, as long as he's all right I'll fit something in to eat. (9, p. 37)

Parents felt guilty simply having gone for a cup of tea or coffee. Such was the desire and pressure that parents experienced to be with their child at all times, that taking a break could feel almost like an act of abandonment. As this mother explained:

I mean, you wouldn't be in the house and walk out to a cafe for an hour and leave your child unattended in the house, so you don't do it in the hospital. (Mother 5, 26, p. 82)

This mother's reference to her child being left 'unattended' highlighted what parents felt was one of the most valued services that could have been provided. What was wanted was a nurse to offer to relieve them and to watch over or sit with their child while they went for their break or meal. This seemed to be a rare occurrence, however, as these parents noted during a focus group interview:

Mother 5: Nobody has said, 'When you want to go for your lunch, give us a shout and we'll watch your child for you.' . . . nobody's actually said that they will do it and you feel obliged because you're their mother.
PD: Would you like someone to come up and say, 'Look, away for your dinner and I'll stay with. . .?
Mother 2: Oh aye! I'd love that.
Mother 4: That would be great.

Parents often found it difficult to ask permission to leave the ward for a break lest this was seen by others as a dereliction of duty:

> They knew you were travelling but nobody would say, 'Away you go and have a cup of tea and we'll watch her,' and I don't feel brave enough to say, 'Can I go?', you know, I felt that I shouldn't. that was one bit that was a bit hard. (12, p. 19)

This highlighted the position of relative powerlessness which parents believed that they occupied. The following parents' comments show that part of their reluctance stemmed from their perceptions of nurses as being forever too busy to undertake such an activity as staying with their child. They also felt that asking for such help might be seen as a personal failing:

> The nurses see me working with her and they see Mr Brown [the child's father] working with her and they say, 'You know, you're coping really great, I don't know where you get all your energy from,' but then sometimes I've got to ask them, Philip, to do it for me and give me a wee break. I find I'm feeding her, changing her, putting her down, sitting her up . . . all the time, and they're short-staffed sometimes . . . can't get a nurse to help you 'cos they're run off their feet. (5, p. 6–7)

> You don't feel like . . . suppose there are six nurses on the ward standing doing nothing, you don't want to go up to them and say, 'Look, would you go in and sit with Alex till I get [while I have] my dinner? (Mother 1, 25, p. 41)

The parents who mentioned that a nurse had offered to sit with their child while they took a break described both surprise and gratitude:

> One morning one of the assistant play leaders came in and said that 'We're really quiet, why don't you go for a walk down to the shops' and she would sit with her for an hour . . . and I really had to force myself [said ironically], I said, 'Oh, great!' (10, p. 22)

Parents were often accurate in their assessment of nurses as being 'rushed off their feet'. The wards were frequently very busy and nurses were engaged in work that, within the context of the ward, would be deemed more important than 'baby-sitting' children whose parents had gone for a break. It would be simplistic, however, to see this as the sole reason for parents' reluctance to ask nurses to watch over their child. In the status hierarchy of work that exists in a paediatric ward (Cleary, 1977; 1979; Brown, 1989), sitting with a child may be viewed as a task of little importance. It is even possible that a nurse who offered to do this might find herself accused of attempting to shirk from some of the 'real work' that needed to be done (Melia, 1987). Likewise, the parents often spoke of how they were reluctant to trouble nurses with 'trivial' matters because this would deflect them from carrying out more important nursing care of children who were more seriously ill. Because of the nature of the treatment of the more seriously ill children, this was usually deemed to be nursing of a more procedural or technical nature.

Here nurses were again confronted with the tension between the individual and universal nature of their work. On one hand their professional ideology was promoting ideas such as individualized and family-centred nursing care. On the other hand, the nurses were aware that more universal concerns meant that they had a responsibility towards not only one child or parent, but to all 20 or 30 in the ward. This tension could confront the nurses with dilemmas that posed the question 'If I do this for one child or parent, will they all want or expect it and, if they do, will I be able to provide it?' To pre-empt this dilemma the nurses tended to politely refuse such requests for individualized services which they believed might set such precedents.

The nurse might also have found that she was making a promise (to sit with or to 'keep an eye on' a child) that she was unable to keep. She might have been asked by a nurse in charge to undertake other duties or might have had to leave the child to respond to the more pressing needs of another. These possibilities were very real, even on wards that claimed to use a system of patient allocation where a nurse had a responsibility for a specific small group of children.

There were also very real organizational problems which prevented nurses from helping parents to take the breaks which they needed so badly. Parents were discouraged from having meals or snacks at the child's bedside, usually for safety reasons. The timing of breaks and meals was the same for both staff and parents. This meant that at the very times when parents needed to be relieved for breaks and meals, the number of available nurses was at its lowest as they too were taking their breaks.

4.2.7 Summary

The parents' descriptions of their participation suggested that this was not so much a deliberate nursing philosophy and strategy as an unspoken and haphazard arrangement. This was more pronounced in relation to the child's everyday rather than technical care, where it was more clear that the demarcation of care made this the nurses' domain unless negotiated otherwise. Parents' accounts also showed that the encouragement of participation seemed to be dependent upon the thoughtfulness of individual nurses who tried to enable and empower parents in ways that were comfortable and acceptable to them.

The participation of parents in their child's care seemed to exist predominantly at the level of the parents carrying out basic mothering work that was viewed merely as a continuation of a mother's normal parenting practices at home. Some parents would become involved in more technical tasks such as nasogastric feeding or suctioning. I argue, however, that the parent's participation could more meaningfully be called the parent's agreement to take over certain tasks from nurses. The parents who seemed to progress to undertaking more technical tasks tended to be the parents of children who required such procedures to be performed over a lengthy period of time, for example children who were comatose and recovering from serious head injuries. In this context such technical tasks were transformed by their becoming routine and thus they became suitable tasks for parents to undertake.

4.3 NURSES AND THE CREATION OF PARENT PARTICIPATION

This discussion of parent participation has focused primarily on the parents. However, as I wish to show that social phenomena within the paediatric ward are co-created by the respective participants, it is now appropriate to consider in more detail the perspectives of the nurses.

Chapter 1 showed that previous research literature has tended to focus exclusively upon nurses' attitudes towards the concepts of parental involvement and participation. It seemed to have been largely accepted that parental participation was an occupational reality which nurses could either be for or against.

Little consideration has been given to how paediatric nurses perceive the meaning of many of the phrases currently being used to encapsulate this notion of parental participation. 'Encourage parents to participate in their child's care' is but one of the expressions that has entered paediatric nursing discourse, that has profound implications for paediatric nursing practice but that has remained relatively unexplored.

In this section I draw predominantly on nurses' accounts to illustrate how the process of parent participation was created, especially from the nurses' perspective. This involves examining more fully the nurses' influence in shaping the extent and nature of parent participation and the nurses' understandings of the value of this arrangement.

I also explore further how the phenomenon of parent participation came about largely as an unspoken agreement, but now looking more from the nurses' perspective. In doing so I examine the strategies that nurses described when they encouraged parents to participate. Finally, I briefly investigate the particular impact that parent participation had upon the nurse–parent–child relationship and upon parent's and nurses' respective power and status. I illustrate this using the example of nurses' accounts of their dealings with what I have termed 'expert parents'.

4.3.1 Parent participation: nurses' understandings and practices

In Chapter 2 I described how nurses had particular expectations regarding live-in parents in relation to their co-operation, competence and character. From the nurses' accounts and descriptions of parent participation it seemed that a similar set of expectations were present regarding this particular aspect of living-in. In addition to their first impressions, nurses described other influences on how they assessed a parent's 'readiness' to participate in their child's care. They took readiness cues as being indications upon which to base their assessments of parents' potential participation. This readiness included a consideration of parents' willingness, interest, timing, ability and the nature of the task in which the parent may have been expected to become involved.

Nurses were sensitive to the importance of timing in their attempts to encourage parent participation. The nurses spoke of assessing parents' readiness to participate in care in ways that indicated that there was a temporal element to participation and that timing was important for parents if they were to be successfully helped to participate. For example if a child had been admitted as an emergency to an intensive care unit, the severity of his illness or injury combined with the unfamiliarity of the surroundings would adversely affect the parents' readiness to help in his care. This did not suggest an unwillingness but illustrated that the parents' anxiety and dread would mean that the time would not be right for them to actively assist in care. The nurses' understandings of readiness suggested that parents needed time to adjust to each change in their child's condition and that they first had to accommodate such changes before moving on. One nurse described how she assessed and interpreted this lack of readiness in parents:

PD: What sort of things do you notice and pick up about parents that help you to make that decision [regarding which parents she would encourage to participate]? . . . Can you think of an example?
Nurse D: Parents that run a mile when the doctors come to take blood, and immediately hand over their child at **any** procedure. I think they are the ones who take a bit longer to . . . you know . . . not that they're not capable but just that either they're frightened or they don't have the confidence. (31, p. 6–7)

This nurse brought out the temporal feature of this readiness by acknowledging that this was not synonymous with lack of capability and that parents could not call forth this participation until they felt ready within themselves.

A nurse from the burns and plastic surgery unit described this temporal aspect of readiness in terms more resonant with meaningful participation when she spoke of how she gauged parents' readiness by the extent of their acceptance or non-acceptance of the child's condition. For this nurse, it was important that parents and nurse shared a similar understanding, of the nature and implications of the child's condition before any meaningful participation could be negotiated. This nurse felt that discrepant perspectives here would nullify any attempts that she might have made to involve or specifically teach the parent.

Up the stairs [in the burns and plastic surgery unit] it's like, your initial . . . it's the way they react to the initial injury that makes you think, right, they've accepted this and this is how they go on from here. If they've got problems grasping, like, what's happened and why it's happened you then have a problem that you can't . . . because they haven't understood what's happened, you can't teach them something to put an input into what you're trying to do. (30, Nurse C, p. 9)

Another nurse described the importance of this timing in ensuring that parents were not 'forced' beyond their own sense of readiness:

There are some parents you think, oh well, maybe that is beyond them . . . so then you won't force that issue, as yet . . . perhaps in a wee while, but not in the beginning, 'cos you don't honestly think that they're ready for it. (30, Nurse B, p. 6)

In assessing if and when parents were to be encouraged to participate, it has already been shown that nurses set great store by their initial and intuitive judgements. For them, first impressions were important. When nurses replied to questions in this way I asked them to try to think of any specific parental cues that might have influenced them as they made these initial assessments. The nurses looked for signs that parents were willing as well as ready to participate in their child's care. As this nurse noted:

I think a lot depends on the parent, if they're willing, you know, you chat to them, and mention, 'Would you like to help do this?' . . . and some are very apprehensive and just don't want to. (29, Nurse C, p. 11)

Parents showed such willingness by directly offering to help and by asking if they could carry out particular tasks. This was also shown more subtly by perhaps asking where the nappies were kept or whether they might have a clean bath towel. One nurse described this:

I suppose if they start asking, 'Can I do that?' you obviously say, 'Certainly' or 'We'd rather we did it' or something like that. I think if they start saying something like, 'I feel a bit helpless, you know, can I help? Can I do something?' Obviously you would let them do something. (1, p. 5)

The nurses also interpreted parents' questioning as being an indication of willingness to participate. As this nurse explained:

I think it's the interest that they show when you're doing something, like if they're . . . say you're putting on a head bandage or something, and you're bandaging him up, if they're, like, having a good look and quizzing you about how you do it, you can then think, well . . . maybe they are capable of doing this, we'll let you try it. (24, p. 6)

The nurses spoke of how they also based their judgements of parents' ability to participate on their perceptions of the parents' competence. One nurse explained how she expected parents to be able to demonstrate their competence in a particular task:

When they come in, if they're interested enough and want to know why you're doing things and are prepared to listen and prepared to give you an example of them doing that then you're quite happy, then I would go ahead and let them. (11, p. 6)

There were both general and particular aspects which nurses took to be indicative of parents' competence and consequently of their ability to participate in their child's care. Nurses noted the parent's general level and style of interaction with their child. As this nurse remarked, '. . . just sort of, maybe, how they generally handle the child . . . ' (23, Nurse I, p. 5). Another nurse gave a more detailed account of this:

I think a lot of it is experience . . . it seems a silly word to put on it at times but I think a lot of it is, you seem to just know inside what parents can do more . . . what parents you can get to . . . what parents you can encourage and what others you're going to help a lot. I mean, I might not have known at first, a few years ago, but now you can more or less sense in the parents how much they want to do and also if they've been doing a lot and when they're getting tired of doing everything then it's time for you to step in again.

PD: Can you think what kinds of things it is, can you think of the criteria that you use?. . . Could you put your finger on them and say that I think about A, B, C and D and that tells me. . . ?

Nurse: Not really, it's quite difficult; maybe the way they handle their own child, whether or not they seem very close to it and want to be with it, whether perhaps they sit away from the bedside, you can sort of see initially whether . . . you know, they want to be there but don't really want to do much with them. (7, p. 6–7)

It seemed from these accounts that assessing parents was largely intuitive and not part of a discourse where nurses were comfortable in attempting to articulate their practice. This is a difficulty clearly recognized in the literature on intuition in nursing (Agan, 1987; Benner and Tanner, 1987).

The general aspects of the parent's approach to the child that were considered valuable indicators of their ability to participate were their expressed care and love for their child. Conversely, parents who seemed distant from their child, due to either less emotionally intense contact or a physical distancing such as 'sitting away from the bed', were seen as being less likely to be able to participate.

When asked if they could describe any specific parental factors that influenced their perceptions of parents' ability to participate, the nurses spoke of the importance of parents' giving the impression of understanding:

The ones that understand what you're doing, you know, if you're trying to explain something and the parents don't seem to be taking it in then there's no use asking them to do a certain procedure or wanting them to help because they'll just not know if they're doing wrong or what they're doing. (7, p. 7)

> If you've been explaining everything to them, how they've taken in the explanations, whether they're maybe too upset, if it's an emergency admission and they're too upset to listen properly, or just intelligence level ... their understanding of the situation. (16, p. 3)

These accounts suggested that nurses assessed parents' ability to participate partly on how parents responded to the nurse's professional interpretation and explanation of the situation. How could a parent show an understanding of the situation that would satisfy nurses that they were capable of participation?

Parent participation seemed to be shaped and determined by a dynamic process involving both parents and nurses. The nurses tended to make their assessments of parents' readiness, willingness and ability to participate in their child's care on the basis of largely unarticulated intuitive responses to general cues and impressions given by parents. In this respect, nurses seemed to positively assess parents who showed obvious love and concern for their child as expressed through close physical contact and caring handling.

Nurses similarly assessed parents positively who showed keenness and interest in participating by either asking directly to do so or by hovering interestedly beside the child while the nurse was carrying out some aspect of the child's care. By doing this it was more likely that the nurse would then ask the parent if they would like to help. The influence of the child should not be overlooked, however, as their insistence that the parent was to stay with them and help with any particular care task also had an influence upon a parent's decision to participate.

The nurses described how they assessed which parents they thought most suitable to participate in care. Underlying this activity was the assumption that this participation had some value, either for the child, his parents, the nurse herself or indeed for all concerned with the hospitalization. I therefore asked the nurses about any benefits that they felt had accrued from having parents participating and whether they felt that there were any disadvantages in this.

The nurses often claimed that it was valuable to have close contact with parents as they were the experts, the people who knew their child best. Similarly in their accounts of what they saw as advantages and disadvantages of parent participation, the nurses spoke of how they valued this expertise in terms of what the parents did for their child that might have been more difficult and time-consuming for the nurse. For example, nurses explained this in relation to how parents helped to monitor their child's clinical condition:

> They tend to notice sooner if their child isn't the normal or if they're not acting normally or they're not taking their fluids as well as they normally do.... They know their normal a lot better, although we know a basic normal, they know their own child's normal. (Nurse E, 29, p. 15)

Another nurse described the value of parents in helping with feeding and relieving their child's distress:

They know what their kids eat, they can shut them up when they're crying. (Nurse A, 20, p. 2)

This nurse described how parents' particular knowledge of their child was valued as an individualistic adjunct to the nurse's generic knowledge. As was suggested earlier, it seemed that such parental knowledge was valued, not only for itself but for how it could benefit the nurses through reducing their workload.

4.3.2 Parent participation and the demarcation of care

There were aspects of the child's care that were, at least initially, deemed to be the distinct province of either nurses or parents. Typically, as was shown earlier, this demarcation of work involved the parents being expected and possibly encouraged to do the basic mothering tasks while the more technical tasks remained the preserve of nurses. Nurses described their understandings of this demarcation:

As far as the, sort of, condition is, I mean the normal things that they would do at home . . . the mothering-type things like washing and bathing . . . feeding, nothing medical like giving medicines or anything like that. (Nurse B, 31, p. 1)

I just assume that there's the child, they're going to come in and look after them, well, what I mean looking after them is changing them, washing them and feeding them, that's all I expect of them. (. . .) There is a clear line, likes of dressings and that is what nurses should do for a child 'cos we need to observe what's happening. (21, p. 13, 15)

Well, all their basic things, their feeding, hygiene, is something that mums have been carrying out properly at home, so allowing them to carry on that. (. . .) Observations, things like that is always . . . Why can't a mother take a temperature? . . . that's difficult . . . we seem to draw the line at anything, I suppose, that's technical. (11, p. 7)

This segmentation of work reflected the traditional concept of nurses' work as being concentrated on technical and procedural tasks (Hawthorne, 1974; Melia, 1987). It also suggested that nurses saw little difference between the performance of basic mothering tasks within the home and within the ward. Nurses' reasoning seemed to be that if parents were able to carry out those tasks at home, then they would be able to carry them out equally well while the child was in hospital. Such a perception however, ignored the possibility that I have previously raised, that the meaning of such tasks altered radically for parents within the different context of the ward.

The nurses' accounts of both their work and that of the parents in the ward suggested that they saw a qualitative difference between the basic mothering tasks and the more technical and procedural work. Basic mothering tasks were perceived as being those that essentially anyone could do, since they were no more than an extension of parents' everyday child-care work at home. This idea was expressed by nurses who attempted to minimize the strangeness of the parents' new situation by telling them essentially to 'just do what you would do at home'. A nurse described this:

> If the parents are in I tend to just say, 'Do what you like with the feeds, do what you would do at home, just feed them when you want 'cos you're going to be here to do it anyway so it's no problem'. (Nurse C, 31, p. 17)

Technical tasks, however, were seen as being more problematic and more important. This was reflected in the fact that it was predominantly such technical information that was given the status of being recorded in nursing notes and medical records.

In maintaining such compartmentalization of work, nurses may have been attempting to preserve and protect what they saw as being an exclusive and valued part of their nursing role and function. Dividing work into basic mothering for parents and technical tasks for nurses allowed the nurse to see her role in terms of clearly defined tasks. This distinguished and separated her from parents but, ironically, this could also separate her from the children. If a clearly held family-care perspective was absent, the child alone could become the nurse's central focus, but such a focus tended only to be brought to bear when the need for some technical care arose. Nurses explained how it occurred that children were 'overlooked' and left to their mothers unless requiring some special and usually technical care:

> I suppose as a nurse you do think that, when the mum's there, that's it, you don't really think of the child as much, unless the child's needing **special nursing care** [my emphasis]. (21, p. 2–3)

> If we're very busy and the child isn't needing any **special care** and the mum's living-in and doing all the care, then the nurses basically aren't doing a lot' [my emphasis]. (3, p. 6)

While such demarcation of care was undoubtedly present, the dynamics of the situation between parents and nurses ensured that the potential existed whereby changes and developments could take place in this area of participation. Nurses and parents described how changes in the relationship between them could occur when parents were resident for longer periods of time. Here, a more involved and connected relationship than that of nurse–parent could develop. Within such a changing and, as was suggested by both nurses and parents, improving relationship, it was possible that the previously described demarcation lines could be significantly blurred. I describe these developing relationships in more detail in the following chapter.

4.3.3 Nurses and the unspoken arrangement

The nurses shared the parents' perception that participation was indeed an arrangement that was rarely discussed at the start of the hospitalization. Not only was this rarely discussed among nurses and parents but some of the nurses commented that this seemed to them to be a strange question and one which they had 'never really thought about before'. I argue that what was largely an unspoken agreement for parents was similarly so for nurses.

The nurses generally agreed that discussion with parents concerning participation did not take place at the outset of their stay, although some felt that this was something that should occur.

> I think it's bad when parents do come in, I don't think we lay down to them what we are expecting of them (. . .) and I don't always think that they are told exactly what we are expecting from them. (Nurse B, 30, p. 2)

> We expect them to carry on their daily care, like their usual basic care, washing them, feeding them . . . and basically you expect them to do it, but it's never said to them. (24, p. 1)

The nurses seemed to view any developing parental participation as being dependent on the developing relationship that the parents had with ward staff, rather than as the result of any clearly explained guidelines or procedure. The individual nurse was therefore expected to anticipate and to be attuned to possibilities for participation. This was achieved by monitoring and interpreting parental cues which might have signalled the parent's desire or willingness to participate, or to participate more fully. As this nurse explained:

> It takes a very clever nurse to anticipate, does this mum want to be completely involved, partly involved or hardly involved? – say in the first instance, when the child comes back from theatre . . . . . . it's really difficult. (19, p. 3)

Although the nurses' accounts seem to suggest that parent participation was simply something that happened in the absence of any negotiation, it would be inaccurate to imply that nurses took no part in the shaping of the participation process. Nurses described two principal strategies employed in order to allow or encourage parents to participate. These strategies emphasized the common nursing perspective that participation was a gradual process whose pace was largely determined by parents themselves. This contrasts with the parents' perspective described earlier, where they felt that their participation was more under the control of nursing staff.

(a) The inform-and-leave strategy

The nurses described an inform-and-leave strategy where they gave parents what they felt to be sufficient information and encouragement to allow them to participate in part of their child's care if they so wished. Nurses described how this was done:

> It's very much, 'There's the locker, the nappies are in there and the towels in there and just get on with it.' (Nurse B, 30, p. 2)

If the mum's are there it's 'Here's the bottle, here's the food; do you want to do it?' and you do it as the situation arises rather than beforehand. (16, p. 4)

The nurses presumed that what they were doing was helping parents by allowing them to help using minimum pressure. Implicit within this strategy was the sense that this allowed the parents the option of being able to help with the child's care if they wished to or felt ready to. However, as the earlier discussion of parents' experiences of participation showed, parents felt under pressure to participate in care and to establish their identity as a good, useful and willing worker.

There was a tension apparent in the accounts of the nurses as they described this gradual and seemingly *laissez-faire* approach to encouraging participation. For while they emphasized their wish to allow parents to participate at their own pace and as they wished, they were also clear that such participation was assuredly expected from parents. Such participation might even be viewed as almost a condition of the parents' living-in. As these nurses explained:

If they're there for a large chunk of the day, resident-wise, we expect them to be there, and you expect them to, eventually, to take over from what you start to do. (16, p. 2)

We seem to expect that they will, if they're going to stay, help with the care. (. . .) You expect from the fact that they're staying in that they will do some of the care, that they're not just going to sit there and be bystanders. (7, p. 32)

A similar discordance seemed to characterize the nurses' understandings of how parents should participate in basic mothering as opposed to more technical tasks. The previously discussed aspects of timing, readiness and ability did not seem salient in relation to what was considered to be the more routine of the child's care tasks.

Parent participation was expected in basic mothering care. It seemed to be taken as given by the nurses that this was work which parents could and should begin to undertake shortly after the child's admission or soon after the need for any form of intensive care or demanding medical treatment had passed. One nurse explained that such participation in the child's basic care was indicative of normal parental responsiveness and that, consequently, its absence could be an indication of some pathological problem in the child–parent relationship. As this nurse observed:

That's why they're there, I mean it's their child, even though they're in hospital. They would have to feed it at home. . . . I mean, you could have a six-week-old baby and if Mum's sitting there and the nurse is feeding it you'd think there was something far wrong here. (8, p. 6)

The nurses seemed unaware that the tensions between the inform-and-leave strategy and their expectations regarding parents' participation could create problems for parents. As was revealed in the parents' accounts of participation, they often interpreted such a nursing approach as meaning that they had simply been left to their own devices. They saw their situation as being one where they had to fend for themselves and to learn what they could and could not do by trial and error, usually the latter. This strategy created a consequent problem for parents by placing them in the position where they were the ones expected to make approaches and requests to nursing staff. Nurses seemed to interpret this positively as being synonymous with parents deciding upon their own extent and rate of participation. Parents, however, interpreted it more negatively. They described how this made them seem demanding or a nuisance, through having to regularly ask nurses for permission or assistance.

(b) The as-if-at-home analogy

Nurses also described how they tried to promote participation by encouraging parents to feel more at home. This was usually done by explaining to parents that they should feel free to do whatever they did for the child at home.

I interpret this strategy in two ways. I believe that it was a well-meaning attempt by some nurses to try to minimize for parents the strangeness of their new situation. It also seemed to be an attempt to defuse or minimize any anxieties related to participating that parents might have had by likening their participation in hospital to the everyday care with which they would be familiar at home. Another possible interpretation, however, is that this was a way in which nurses made more explicit to parents the notion that within the ward there was parental work and nurses' work. This would carry the hidden implication that by saying 'Just do whatever you would do at home', nurses were also implying, 'Don't do any other things with your child, because that is our work'. This would also suggest that, while parent participation was still largely an unspoken arrangement, some aspects of the demarcation of nurses' and parents' responsibilities were made explicit. Several nurses described their use of the as-if-at-home analogy:

I expect them to take care of the non-nursing duties of the child, like, you know . . . the feeding, changing, bathing and things like that, obviously, 'cos that's what they would do at home. (21, p. 8)

As far as the, sort of, condition is, I mean the normal things that they would do at home . . . the mothering-type things, like washing and bathing, feeding. . . . (Nurse B, 31, p. 1)

If the parents are in I tend to just say, 'Do what you like with the feeds; do what you would do at home.' (Nurse C, 31, p. 17)

Nurses, however, seemed unaware of the difficulties which parents faced as they tried to sustain this as-if-at-home analogy within the different context of the ward. One illustration of this difficulty has already been given in Chapter 2's discussion of parental disciplinary styles. There, parents found it very difficult to simply 'do what they would do at home'. Similarly, for example in the case of certain burned children, their parents could not simply wash and change them as they would have done at home because the nature and meaning of the injury had rendered this formerly straightforward care problematic.

A further illustration of the difficulty that parents experienced in trying to participate in terms of both the as-if-at-home analogy and the inform-and-leave strategies was revealed, once again, in their accounts of how they had tried to use ward kitchens. I had considered initially that the kitchen may have represented what Goffman termed 'a back region or backstage', an area where there would be 'no audience present' (Goffman 1959, p. 114–115) or, in this case, no parents. However, from my own paediatric nursing experience and from my observations and conversations during the period of field work, I could find no evidence that the kitchen was used by nurses in this way.

Another interpretation of why parents' access to kitchens was restricted turns on the ward kitchen as being a metaphor for the home. This opens up the possibility that allowing parents unrestricted access to and use of the kitchen would be a logical but unacceptable conclusion of both the inform-and-leave and as-if-at-home approaches. If this were so then it may support the second interpretation of nurses' adoption of the as-if-at-home analogy. It may be that nurses had unstated limitations in mind when they encouraged parents to 'just carry on as normal' and to 'do what you would do at home'.

Parents described how this exclusionary practice confounded some of their attempts to participate in the ways suggested by the as-if-at-home analogy. For example, they were unable to simply go and fetch their child a drink if they were thirsty or to make up their baby's feed or to make their child a slice of toast for supper. In addition to contradicting the image of the ward as home which nurses tried to promote, this practice also placed parents in the uncomfortable position of having to risk the censure of nurses. This occurred if they were caught trying to enter the kitchen unnoticed to quickly get a drink or if they had to ask a nurse to do this for them and therefore undertake what the parents saw as a comparatively trivial and nuisance task.

I suggest that the importance of these nursing approaches to encouraging parent participation lies in the unrecognized tension that existed between these articulated strategies and the unspoken expectations that the nurses held. This tension had a direct impact upon parents' lived experience of their participation. For while they received encouragement from nurses that they themselves should determine the nature and extent of their participation by carrying on in ways that were normal for them, there were clearly discernible nursing and institutional expectations and practices which contradicted this seemingly *laissez-faire* approach.

I now take this discussion further by examining the experiences of nurses in relation to a small, but significant group of parents whom I have termed 'expert parents'. These were parents who were expert at managing and 'parenting' their child who had a chronic illness or disability. Their child's health status usually necessitated numerous hospital admissions, either as part of a remission and relapse pattern or for repeated treatment to old injuries.

4.3.4 Nurses and the expert parent

Parental participation influenced the nurse's sense of professional identity. Nurses described a tension wherein they recognized the importance of allowing and encouraging parents to undertake more of their child's care, while also recognizing that this could seem diminishing to their sense of self as nurses. For some nurses, sharing care with and involving parents was not a calling forth of greater connectedness with a whole family. Rather, it seemed that, by 'handing over' aspects of care that had traditionally been viewed as theirs, nurses then saw nothing of comparable value with which to replace them.

This was especially clearly illustrated in the accounts of a nurse who described her relationship with two parents, each of whom she regarded as being an expert parent. One mother had been in the ward for several weeks before the nurse arrived and was carrying out all of her child's care herself. Here she described how she felt that she was no longer 'needed' by this mother:

Nurse: This woman didn't know us [this refers to herself and the other nurse who was participating in the same interview], she didn't need our help, because the acute stage had passed and she could do all this child's care herself now, so she didn't really need us. She's a nice pleasant woman but I haven't got a relationship with her at all, just say, 'Hiya,' and that's it, 'cos she didn't need us.
PD: That's interesting'.
Nurse: No, she doesn't, apart from to help lift or something . . . and plus the wee girl doesn't trust the nurses to lift her as much as her mum anyway. I think when parents have been in a lot longer (. . .) people need you in the acute phase, they don't really need you in the post-acute phase. (Nurse A, 20, p. 53–54)

The nurse also described her relationship with another expert parent, 'Mrs Blue'. This mother had a young teenage child who was very severely disabled as a result of a disorder that had necessitated his having numerous hospital admissions for reconstructive plastic surgery and other treatments. His skin was particularly liable to blister and break down if he was not extremely carefully handled. This section of the nurse's account followed on from a more general discussion of the power and control, or as she perceived it, the lack of power and control that parents had over the course of their child's care and treatment within the hospital.

Nurse: The only person I would say is in any control of her child's life is Mrs Blue, Sam's mother 'cos she knows more about it [Sam's disease] than any of the doctors or nurses and she is the **only** one, and she tells them straight, if a doctor does something or goes near Sam with a needle, she'll say, 'You're not doing that!' ... and they listen to her ... because ... she's the only person I've ever met that has any control over her son's treatment'.

PD: That's fascinating!

Nurse: 'cos she knows more about it than them and they realize that ...

PD: And they actually defer to her and listen to her?

Nurse: Oh aye! 'cos she was telling me that she brought Sam in here in [names the year] and he was playing with cars, he had toy cars and she went away to get something and came back and Sam was breaking his heart [weeping] ... she says, 'What's wrong?' ... The doctor had taken away his cars so she went to the house officer and said, 'Can I have Sam's cars back?' and he said, 'No, because they're hard, they're metal and he might hurt himself. She says, 'My son has played with toy cars since he was two years old and has never caused a blister' and he said, 'What he may do at home is different from what he may do here, Mrs Blue, and he's not playing with them here.' So she got on the phone to Professor Fawn ... he had referred Sam to get his fingers done, and she said, 'You'll have to come up here,' and he came up and seemingly went through [reprimanded severely] this house officer, and she says that ever since that, they know fine well ... and I was reading in his notes that that professor had written a letter and it said that staff in Ward Y obviously do not appreciate Mrs Blue's help ... or they don't appreciate her knowledge and it's true and the woman was telling the truth, she does know best. (20, p. 62–64)

Apart from its force as a moral tale (Baruch, 1981), this nurse's retelling of Mrs Blue's account offered some valuable insights into the characteristics of the expert parent and suggested how these might influence the parent–nurse relationship. Mrs Blue had immediately established her claim to expertise, not simply by being Sam's mother, nor solely by virtue of her length of experience in the hospital arena, in this case for over 10 years. She was able to invoke her more intimately involved practical contact with Sam as an individual in order to overcome any theoretical or textbook objections and precautions to his playing with toy cars.

She also countered the doctor's attempt to use his abstract hospital-based knowledge to transmute the as-if-at-home analogy into a criticism that would have negated her expertise. As an expert parent she also had an influential contact in the Professor, as indeed many expert parents are likely to have due to their prolonged and regular contact with recognized professional experts in their field. She used the elements of her expert status in a way that could have created difficulties for her: by using one health professional to confront and contradict another. The expert parent, however, seemed to have the power, derived from unique and specialist knowledge, and the self-confidence that arose from this to enable her to carry out such an assertive strategy.

It seems understandable, therefore, given the specific knowledge and skilled practices of an expert parent, that a nurse might feel that they had comparatively little to offer to their child. If a nurse were to consider that her professional identity was created solely through the tasks that she carried out, then such parental expertise could effectively deny the nurse the opportunity to be a nurse within those particular narrow terms.

The expert parent is considered to have passed the critical stage of being shocked and overwhelmed by the child's illness or injury. Over time and through experience they may also have developed personally effective coping strategies enabling them to deal with the repeated hospital admissions (Hayes and Knox, 1984; Robinson, 1985; 1987). Being an expert parent calls forth new ways of being with and caring for a child. I suggest also that expert parents may have developed new self-understandings that could lessen their need for nurses or others to provide 'psychological support'. I recall here the parents who described how their lives, their thinking and their values would never be the same. As one mother wrote in her diary:

It takes something like this accident to put things right back into perspective.
Silly trivial things will never bother me again.

The expert parent's self-understandings may in turn have noticeably altered the relationship between the parent and nurse. If the basis of such a relationship was the existence of a professional thought to possess greater knowledge and sought-after skills, and a more vulnerable and dependent party, then the expert parent seemed to have reversed this scenario in relation to both general and specific aspects of their child's care and treatment.

In the case of 'Mrs Blue', she was recognized as having specialist knowledge and skills pertaining to her child; skills and knowledge which the ward professionals had not only to acknowledge but actively draw upon in order to ensure the child's care and treatment within the ward. Consequently, it may have been the nurses who were the vulnerable and dependent parties. Their professional identity had been paradoxically confused, possibly by the success of previous nursing endeavours that stressed the importance of helping parents to cope, encouraging their participation and teaching them the skills needed so that they may be better able to care for their child.

4.4 CONCLUDING COMMENTS

In this chapter I have examined both nurses' and parents' accounts of their experiences related to parent participation within the ward. Interpretive analysis suggested that the concept of parent participation was very much a phenomenon co-created by both nurses and parents. However, there seemed to be significant tensions and incongruities within these respective understandings. For example, nurses had definite but often unexpressed expectations of parents, yet their strategies to encourage participation stressed that participation should be largely determined by parents themselves. The term 'parent participation' seemed to have a meaning for nurses and parents that implied an arrangement where one party, the parents, would be allowed by the other party, the nurses, to help with their child's care. This perception seemed to be underpinned by a view of the nurse–parent relationship that perceived the nurse as being the dominant power figure and the parent as being in a more secondary and compliant role. Within this perspective it seemed more likely to be the nurse who would ultimately decide upon the critical aspects of participation and the parents who would participate accordingly. The impression gained from participants' accounts was of parents as helpers, functioning in a role akin to an unqualified member of the ward staff. The parents' efforts at participation were thus directed towards areas of care that were incidentally if not primarily useful for nurses to have done by others, for example basic mothering.

What seemed to be largely missing from the nurses' and parents' account of participation was any real sense of involvement, reciprocity and mutuality. By this I mean an involvement where parents felt that they had retained an acceptable control over both their own and their child's lives. This involvement would also be characterized by feeling that aspects of both their child's care and their own role were truly negotiable and a proper subject for discussion and genuine dialogue, and where they felt that their participation in the child's care was of worth and value in terms other than those of helping out the nurses. In the absence of such involvement, I argue that the concept of parental participation was more akin to 'parents who stayed for a long time and helped out the staff'. On this subject, one mother made a rueful point.

Father 3: You do feel involved, the things that we do for the bairn . . .
Mother 2: Aye, but we're just visitors to them [the hospital staff]. (25, p. 85)

There was also a tension apparent in that some nurses felt that, by encouraging parents to undertake more of their child's care, they as nurses were consequently diminished. This diminution was not only professional but also emotional and personal in the sense that nurses spoke of no longer 'being needed'. For these nurses it seemed as if encouraging parent participation was not a practice they viewed as being mutually empowering and satisfying but an alienating and exclusionary process that could deprive the nurse not only of contact with parents but, more importantly for them, with the child.

However, there were parents who described their experience of living-in in ways that showed that they had felt valued and useful and that other nurses had enabled them to be meaningfully involved in their child's care. These parents and nurses may well have agreed with Gadamer's insight that:

'Participation' is a strange word. Its dialectic consists of the fact that participation is not taking parts, but in a way taking the whole. Everybody who participates in something does not take something away, so that others cannot have it. The opposite is true by sharing, by our participating in the things in which we are participating, we enrich them they do not become smaller, but larger. (Gadamer 1984, p. 64)

The following chapter will explore the relationships that developed between nurses and parents that could enable such mutual understandings.

ACKNOWLEDGEMENT

This chapter first appeared as Darbyshire, P. (1993) Parents, nurses and paediatric nursing: a critical review. *Journal of Advanced Nursing*, **18**, 1670–80. Reprinted by permission of Blackwell Scientific Publishers Ltd.

5 | Parents' and nurses' relationships

5.1 INTRODUCTION

Describing and exploring the live-in parents' relationships is important for several reasons. A clearer understanding of the concepts of 'family' and 'parent' is contextually dependent. Examination of the parents' relationships can further illuminate the nature of the parents' being-in-the-world (Heidegger, 1962) as live-in parents. The parents' network of relationships is a useful lens through which to view the ways in which parents' social identities are formed within the ward. The parents' relationship network also provides insights into larger theoretical issues, for example the social organization of paediatric nursing and the nature of nursing's central concept, caring (Roach, 1987; Watson, 1988b; Benner and Wrubel, 1989).

5.2 PARENTS' PERCEPTIONS OF NURSES AND NURSING

An important influence on the relationships which developed between nurses and parents was parents' perceptions of the nurse as an individual and of nursing in general. Parents described both individual nurses and their general understandings of nurses' work in response to several different questions raised during our interviews. While most of the parents' accounts arose in response to more direct questions, they also discussed nurses and nursing in connection with other aspects of living-in.

5.2.1 The nurses' work

When describing nurses' work, the majority of parents mentioned the technical or procedural elements such as taking temperatures, pulses and respirations and the basic mothering tasks such as washing, feeding and changing children. These parents' comments were typical:

> They're round checking temperatures and taking their pulse rates, and you see them going back and forth to bring children their feeds and change them and wash them (. . .) and obviously there's times when they go round with the medications too. (9, p. 9–10)

> The nurse takes my child's temperature and pulse and counts his breathing and apart from that, I could honestly say that a nurse has never . . . well . . . they do his dressings (. . .) so they don't actually do anything for him, but then I'm there all the time. (26, Mother 5, p. 31)

> Temperature and pulse, basically; I've seen them coming up sometimes for a bit of a blether, but basically the nurses were there only to take her temperature or her pulse. (12, p. 27)

It is understandable that parents highlighted these aspects of the nurses' work as standing out since nurses checked children's temperature, pulse and respirations at least four times per day. Similarly, basic child-care tasks had to be carried out frequently and again these took place within the main ward. Such activities as recording observations and basic child-care were occasionally seen as being a particularly undemanding and low-level form of nursing, as this parent's comments suggested:

> I think their work must be pretty boring (laughs), that's the idea basically, it doesn't seem particularly skilled work (. . .) it's that it doesn't **look** as if they do particularly much, it's change dressings, give injections and that's it (laughs) . . . but they do have a treatment room which you're not really seeing. (13, p. 26–27)

This mother's point was significant as it acknowledged that there were a great many nursing activities which occurred 'off-stage', which parents might not be aware of and would not have been involved in. Another mother made the point that parents might not have been able to describe what actually constituted nursing work as they themselves were not nurses:

> Aye, but we're not trained nurses, like, to see what they do all day. (25, Mother 2, p. 62)

Parents seemed to accept nursing activities as being simply part of the ward routine rather than as being important interventions which were part of their child's overall care. Paradoxically, they could also be seen as being detrimental to the child's care. One mother described how she saw the performance of routine nursing tasks as something which actually impeded the nurse's ability to be attentive to her restrained child's needs. The child behind the object of their procedures, which the mother saw as being of greater importance, was thus not attended to:

> Nobody was paying attention to him . . . they were going in, taking his temperature, taking his pulse and going out . . . they weren't paying attention, his feet were tied up, see, and his hands were tied up that much that they

were going blue. [This toddler wore arm and ankle restraints postoperatively to prevent him from scratching and destroying his new skin graft.] (15, p. 36–37)

One mother's comments shed light upon an area of difficulty in relation to nurses' work. When parents were asked to discuss nurses and nursing work, they may have limited their responses to what was the most common understanding of the word 'work'. This could also have occurred when less direct questions were used, such as 'Can you tell me how nurses seem to spend their day?' In response to such questions parents may have limited their answers to descriptions of physical work, seeing other non-physical forms of nurses' work as somehow 'not really work' (cf. Melia, 1987). Such a view would be similar to common or lay perceptions of nursing. One mother's comments highlighted this problem well:

PD: That's interesting that you mention physical things like changing dressings . . . what about the sort of non-physical things . . . are you aware of those?

Mother: You mean like talking and things? Oh yes they do.. . . I suppose I tend to think that that's not work 'cos it's quiet, I mean I suppose that's part of the job but you don't consider it as work. (13, p. 27–28)

This perception of nurses' work as being predominantly procedural and physical might account for parents' perceptions of nurses as being almost perpetually busy.

5.2.2 Nurses as perpetually busy

A recurrent theme in the parents' descriptions of nurses and their work was that nurses were invariably very busy, being in almost perpetual motion. Several parents described this:

They're rushing around constantly, they never seem to have the time for any talk to anyone without doing something else, they can't sit and talk to them as such.(. . .) I know what a heavy job they're trying to do and, as I say, they're rushed completely from one thing to another. (4, p. 17)

They're short-staffed sometimes . . . can't get a nurse to help you, you've just got to get on with it 'cos they're run off their feet. (. . .) They'd like to be there longer than what they can but they haven't got the time, they've got to run and do something else. (5, p. 7)

Recall how, in Chapter 3, I suggested that this perception of nurses' perpetual 'busyness' led parents to avoid interrupting nurses for fear of being a nuisance. Parents also felt that nurses were often too busy with children's technical or physical needs to attend to 'less urgent' needs, such as being able to spend time in talking. As these parents explained:

I would say that 80% of them [the nurses] you could have a wee conversation with, but you hate to keep them back from their work 'cos they're aye that busy, so you don't like to talk too long 'cos they're always busy. (28, Mother 4, p. 28)

I know there are children who need feeding, changing, medication that they cannot do, they're totally reliant on the nurses, so they have to go to them and see to their medical needs before they can socialize, but you know ... have five minutes to sit and talk to somebody, they can sit and talk to a baby while they're changing it or feeding it but they can't to John, in that sense, because they sort of think, well, if I [the mother] can get John changed then I [the nurse] can go down and give so-and-so whatever it is. It's not their fault, I don't say they're bad nurses, it's the fact that there's not enough staff for the children to have a little bit of time, not just John but the others as well. It's a case of just see to their needs, put them down and hope they're quiet. (4, p. 15)

This last excerpt was from a mother whose son was 11 years old and was recovering from a head injury but had not yet regained his speech or full mobility. She made the significant point that her son had no pressing physical or technical needs, which she felt led nurses to spend less time with him than with other children whose physical care needs were perhaps greater. She also felt that 'socializing' with her son was an activity which required to be legitimated by doing it under the protective cover of carrying out a concomitant physical activity. The problem was that, unlike babies who required feeding, there was no act of physical care which would give the nurse the justificatory excuse needed to 'socialize' with John.

John's mother explained another common concern related to nurses' busyness. Parents watched nurses carefully to see how they treated children whose parents were not with them. From these impressions they imagined how their child might fare in the ward if they were ever left alone. As one mother explained:

When you're there, they're so kind and gentle and put time in. . . . Are they like that when you're not there or is it all rush and tumble? (4, p. 16)

This point was echoed by another mother who felt that her handicapped baby required a great deal of stimulation while in hospital if he was not to 'go backwards' developmentally. She explained that because her baby was physically handicapped and therefore more passive and undemanding, he would be unable to elicit from others the concentrated caring attention and stimulation which she provided.

They wouldn't hear him crying unless he was crying really sore [hard][the baby was in a ward cubicle], but above these other babies they would never hear him ... but he'd probably get fed and changed and that's him [that would be all]. There'd be very little eye contact 'cos what I do notice is, any nurse feeding any baby, there's very little eye contact ... you watch them with a bottle and they sit there and (gestures looking all around her) ... I've noticed that, so he'd lose out on all that. (6, p. 5)

Nurses' busyness seemed an integral part of the social context of the ward sustained by both parents and nurses. Parents described nurses' busyness in such a way as to suggest that viewing nurses in ways other than being extremely hard-working was almost a betrayal of the nurses' efforts on behalf of their child. Nurses too supported this emphasis on their extreme busyness. It was common to hear competitive stories in the coffee room, where nurses would claim the honour of being in the busiest ward which had been 'going like a fair' or where they had 'never stopped' that morning.

This perception of nurses as perpetually busy with predominantly physical and technical work has been reported by previous researchers (Pill, 1970; Melia, 1987) who suggested that it was an impression deliberately created by nurses in response to the social pressures and unwritten rules of the ward. Similarly, in Menzies's (1967) classic study, it was suggested that nurses' preoccupation with fragmented physical tasks was a defence mechanism which protected them from the stress involved in having to confront a powerful range of emotions, It is tempting to conclude from these parents' accounts that the old nursing adage of 'Always look busy, even when you're not' (cf. Melia, 1987) may have been adhered to, but an alternative explanation is that the nurses were genuinely extremely busy.

The significant question from the perspective of this research was not, however, whether the nurses were 'really' busy or merely conforming to social pressures. What is of greater relevance here are the implications of these perceptions of nurse busyness for the nature of the nurse–parent relationship. One implication is that busyness can become highly prized in its own right and can come to constitute, on its own, normative, valued nursing practice. Thus nurses may attach a disproportionate importance to the speedy completion of physical care tasks, or to the ability to physically 'cope' in the face of greatly increased demands. In such a situation it is possible that the aspects of nursing which cannot, by definition, be hurried, or timed in the way that taking a temperature might take five minutes, will be pushed further down the list of priorities, being seen as activities which do not attract similar kudos to being exceptionally busy.

Significantly, however, parents suggested that it was precisely during such periods of increased busyness and demanding workload that nurses' caring practices could be thrown into the sharpest relief. In this study, I distinguish caring practices from mere behaviours in that practices are socially organized, constituted culturally and have inherent meaning within a context (Taylor, 1985b). Caring practices also have an sense of good embedded within them (MacIntyre, 1981).

The subsequent discussion of nurses finding and taking time will develop this point in more detail. Here, however, two accounts from parents were particularly illustrative of the importance of caring in relation to busyness. One parent was particularly impressed by a nurse who had been extremely busy yet had taken the time to detour from her task in hand to straighten her daughter's pillows and make her more comfortable. Another parent described a nurse as being particularly caring who had taken the time to come from the main ward to the ICU to quickly say that she would try to get a minute to come and see her at some point during her shift.

Taken only as discrete behaviours these events scarcely merit comment. A nurse fixing a pillow and a nurse popping her head momentarily through the door of the ICU seem events of little significance. However, when understood as caring practices, it is clear that these events were deeply valued by parents who saw them as confirmation that the nurse was attentive to their and their child's 'smallest' needs.

Showing through the parents' perceptions of the nurses' busyness is the parents' need for caring both for their child and for themselves, during a time which is widely recognized as being extremely stressful and traumatic. This examination of the nurse–parent relationship offers insights into the nursing approaches and practices which parents experienced as being caring and, conversely, those which provoked more negative feelings and responses.

5.2.3 The value of nurses' caring practices

The parents described a range of encounters in which they felt that a nurse had made a positive or valued intervention with either their child or themselves. Parents valued nurses who were patient and unhurried in their interactions with parents and children; nurses who 'took the time' or 'found the time' to speak to parents or to do something seen as special for the child. One mother described how two staff nurses had coaxed her reluctant daughter into taking her medicine:

> They tried to coax her for 10 minutes to take this medicine, and she was crying and she hadn't even tasted it, she just didn't want to take it and they stood very patiently and said, 'Alice, it'll make you feel better and. . .' . . .and I thought after that, what patience! [. . .] They **spent time** you know, they didn't give you a minute and then force it, they gave time . . . patience. (14, pp. 16–17)

This 'taking time' was also described by other mothers:

> Sally [a student nurse] is awfully good with her. She'll sit and talk to her, play with her, get her teddies and play with her and she'll sit her up or she'll fix her pillows . . . you don't get many nurses that'll do that, Philip, 'cos they've not got the time, but she picks time to do it, she'll say, 'Away you go for a cup of tea and I'll play with her for a wee while.' (5, p. 10)

Unhurried approaches were also appreciated where nurses were seen to be responsive and understanding towards children whose behaviour was regarded, even by parents, as bad. As one mother explained:

> I found that the nurses on our ward have got a lot more patience with the children than I would ever have, 'cos a lot of them on our ward at the moment need their backsides smacked, and the way that they can still speak

to them nicely and still get them what they want after they've been sworn at and all sorts . . . it amazes me. I think the ones we've got just now are really good. (26, Mother 5, p. 64)

Nurses 'taking time' for parents and children confirmed for parents that they were not merely names on a Kardex or bodies in a bed. Through nurses' focused attention, parents and children were acknowledged and respected as persons in an environment where depersonalization and alienation were very real possibilities.

Parents also valued nurses whose caring practices allowed them to talk about what was of importance to them and to express their feelings openly. These nurses genuinely and actively listened and heard in an accepting and non-judgemental way. Two parents explained this:

I suppose that it's somebody that doesn't mind me talking and mentioning all the things and somebody who explains everything to me (. . .) they would say, 'Don't be embarrassed, just if you want to cry just sit there and cry 'cos you have to get it out.' (17, p. 22, 39)

Staff Nurse Patricia was the first one I'd say that came and spoke to me, and she said to me, 'What do you think of him?' and I says, 'I think it's great, but if he could just get out of here [the ICU]. . . ' and she says, 'Well, it's just going to take a lot of time.' She never says a lot, but she helps you that wee bit, you know, there's folk that you speak to and you feel a wee bit better afterwards – I felt a wee bit better. (18, p. 34–35)

Nurses who were warm and friendly were also appreciated and often sought out by parents. These comments were typical of this:

If there's a friendlier approach you appreciate it more. You're a person then, not just **this mother, a parent**. (13, p. 29)

The nurse that is pregnant is very nice in many ways and I really felt at ease with her (. . .) just her general approach was so warm . . . so nice. (9, p. 26)

Nurses who were warm and friendly not only helped parents on an individual level but helped to create a more accepting and relaxed healing climate (Benner, 1984). Within such a community of caring, parents could more easily make the transition from normal parenting to parenting under stress and under public and professional scrutiny. Parents made a special mention of nurses who 'showed an interest' in both themselves and their child. This seemed to be a way of describing nurses who were alert and vital in their interactions with the families. This was in contrast to those nurses who may have carried out similar work but who were perceived to be merely 'going through the motions'. Two mothers described their experience with nurses who 'took an interest':

Two different nurses really made a point of either spending a bit of their time coming and talking to him and doing things, or they'd either . . . one of them particularly went, I think she said she would like to feed him so she fed him and then got him changed and ready for bed and another one did much the same thing for me and they were saying what had happened with the tests and drugs and things like that, just showing interest more than anything. (2, p. 39–40)

They took an interest. I mean there's ones that can stand and blether [gossip] to you, I don't mean that kind (. . .) but the nurses that have took an interest in Alan, have seen to him, that have went over and spoke to him, **they spoke**, they've actually took time and spoke, and said well, he's there, he's a live person, it's him that's in here not just the mum, it's him.. . . 'Hello, wee man,' you know, and just spoke. [Note that this baby had a congenital chromosomal abnormality that had resulted in a limb deformity.] (6, p. 18)

This mother nicely differentiated between 'just blethering' and 'taking an interest'. While general conversation with nurses was often valued as a distraction, this was not the same as nurses taking a real interest in the child. Taking an interest showed a sense of purpose on the part of the nurses who had been closely involved in his care through 'seeing to him' and who had allowed the baby behind the handicap to show up.

Parents valued nurses whose caring practices acknowledged their own needs as well as their child's. A mother who had been unwell described how nurses showed concern for her when she returned to the ward:

When I came down about two hours later [from her room] there were about three nurses came up and asked how I was and you know, if I wasn't feeling too good just to go and tell them (. . .) and you know it was lovely, 'cos, you know, it was just a bit of caring, just a nice thought really for them to come and ask, 'cos they needn't have done . . . just a bit of interest as well, isn't it?. (2, p. 23–24)

Nurses who took an interest in both the parents and the child helped to establish a sense of connectedness between themselves, the child and the parents. I use the expressions 'connection' and 'connectedness' in a dual and more phenomenological sense to include not only initial meetings and interactions but a sense of mutuality and involvement where the evolution of shared understandings and purposes continued to develop throughout the parent's stay. Morse (1991, p. 458) also describes such connected relationships as 'viewing the patient (*sic*) first as a person and second as a patient, while maintaining a professional perspective'. One mother explained this concisely when she observed that 'some of these nurses, they just click' (27, Mother 4, p. 53).

Such connectedness with nurses enabled parents to share and validate their concerns and problems. When such connectedness was not established and maintained, there seemed a greater likelihood that parents' sense of isolation and exclusion could be heightened. This was exemplified in the accounts of parents who described their experience of hospitalization in terms of how 'No one really understands what this is like'.

Another theme that ran through parents' positive descriptions of nurses and their caring practices was their appreciation of those nurses who supported and coaxed them, fostering hope through encouragement. One father's account of his son's serious scalding and subsequent period in the intensive care unit was notable for the frequency of references that he himself made to encouraging his son to fight for his life. This father particularly appreciated nurses who shared his sense of fighting optimism:

> I was just crying at the cot there and holding his hand and praying and say-ing to him, 'Fight it!' and the nurse that was there, she comforted me and says, 'Just keep hoping and it'll be all right; he's going to be all right.' (18, p. 55–56)

Another mother felt that she had gained strength from the nurses who were so supportive towards her and who had really 'got behind' her baby in his fight:

> There are certain nurses who have cared for him quite often and I feel really care about him . . . not, obviously, as much as I do but who are really behind him.(. . .) Basically they keep your spirits up, they've kept mine up (. . .) they do jolly me along. (17, p. 22)

Throughout the parents' accounts of their valued experiences of nurses and their caring practices I gained the impression that these instances were thought by the parents to be exceptional. To the parents, they seemed to represent nursing that was somehow above and beyond what they might have reasonably expected. Parents were pleasantly surprised when, for example, a nurse who had perhaps been moved to another ward would return to see their child or to ask how they were getting on:

> The ones that have been shifted come up from other wards to see him, so it makes us feel good, kenning [knowing] that they care. (18, p. 63–64)

> Even the ones that are in different wards, if they see me walking up and down with the bairn they'll come up and ask how he's getting on and that, it's been really great. (15, p. 21)

Similarly, parents expressed surprise when nurses 'went out of their way' to do something 'exceptional' for them or their child:

> I found that they try their best to make you feel homely, like . . . they'll go out of their way to . . . at the start we were a bit funny about what Sally could eat, you know, and they came up and were asking us and no matter what we said, they would go out of their way to get that for us, you know, so I found that nice, you know, I just found it reassuring. (12, p. 11)

> There was one on the day that was awfully nice to the wee one. She said,

'How would you like me to go and get you a nice drink of milk and a biscuit?' 'cos they've been trying to get him to drink . . . . He thought that was great! I thought it was thoughtful 'cos nobody else had done that for him. (28, Mother 4, p. 28–29)

Two parents commented on nurses who had given of their own time, over and above their allocated span of duty:

There was another student who worked on the first bad day and I'll never forget that 'cos she was sitting her Highers but she spent that day when they thought that he had brain damage . . . she was here an extra hour, that's bar her nine hours . . . she was an awfully good nurse. (18, p. 39)

Like today, there was one nurse who was actually off duty and there was Jill and another little boy and she had bought a video and crisps and things . . . Jill was asleep, as it happened, but she took the little boy to her flat . . . that's how good they are.

These nurses gave more of themselves than their contracted hours and were willing to make more of a commitment to the children and their parents. This was also a good example of the point made by Gadow (1980), Benner and Wrubel (1989) and others, that the professional and the personal qualities of the nurse cannot be artificially separated as they are inextricably bound together.

Parents valued other caring practices. They appreciated being allowed to speak freely and to be carefully listened to. They appreciated being allowed to express their emotions in an accepting and non-judgemental atmosphere and to have matters relating to their child's care and treatment explained to them in a way that they could understand. They appreciated nurses who were genuinely interested in them and in their child and who expressed this interest through a warm, friendly and unhurried relationship. They appreciated being involved in their child's care but also being offered choices as to what they wished to do or not to do. They appreciated having their needs as parents recognized and responded to, and not only those of their child. However, there were also occasions when the relationship between parents and nurses was strained and characterized not by caring and mutuality but by distrust, dissatisfaction and anger.

5.2.4 The absence and breakdown of caring practices

Parents' descriptions of encounters with nurses that they found to be unsatisfactory reflected the converse of those previously described. They complained of nurses who were overbearing or bossy, who seemed to have no time for children or parents, who talked down to them 'as if they were stupid' or, alternatively, who discussed matters in terms that the parents could not understand.

Parents were very sensitive to both the content of what was being said and also how it was being said. They were quite certain that they had not misinterpreted when they had been spoken to rudely and in ways that fostered a sense of alienation from their child's care. The following parents' accounts illustrated this clearly:

> I could have got really annoyed at the way she [the nurse] spoke to the wife [my wife] about it . . . 'cos she was awfully abrupt, ken [you know], she was right [very] straightforward, and it was just as well she stopped when she did, 'cos if she'd have carried on then I was actually going to tell her what I thought . . . which wouldn't have been very nice. (12, p. 6–7)

> Well, I was standing outside the cubicle with Sean in my arms and she [the nurse] came up and said, 'I'll give you a tip, just **stay in** the cubicle with Sean,' as all the other children had viruses of sorts. (. . .) I was standing outside the cubicle in a bit of a dream because I'd been told that Sean was having his barium meal and it really set my mind going and I was upset and when she said that it made me 10 times worse and I almost began to cry when she said that. . . . If she'd just came up and said to me, 'I'd rather if you didn't mind staying in the cubicle', that was all. (9, p. 27–28)

> There was one day he fell and the bandage went back and I went to see her [the nurse] and I said, 'Could you take a look at Ben's head or change his bandage?' (mimics nurses sarcastic voice) 'Oh dear what a shame!' . . . and she walked away . . . and I went, 'Hey! Come back!' . . . I was angry. . . . It wasn't what she had said but the way she had said it, it wasn't, 'Oh what a shame' said with concern. (15, p. 38–39)

Parents were critical of nurses' actions that fostered their sense of aloneness and exclusion from their child's care. Their accounts of 'being ignored' revealed that this was a source of much anger and resentment.

> He threw up all over me 'cos he choked on a lump and there's no one there to help you with it. . . . I'm sitting with a knee full of sick, a baby covered in sick, a bowl in one hand, it was on the floor, on the buggy, **everywhere** . . . and the nurses walked past. But if **they** had been feeding him and he had been sick, another nurse would have come and helped them to clean it up. (26, Mother 5, p. 25–26)

> You feel as though they're neglecting your child . . . they're not, but in a way they are to you because nobody's spending any time with him (. . .) and I keep thinking, well, nobody's bothering at all here. . . . You're not important as such. (4, p. 21)

> You're sitting there bubbling and greeting [weeping] . . . and they're going by you . . . even if they'd said, 'Look, come on and we'll take you down and buy you a wee cup of tea' or something, but **nothing** . . . they just walk by you and kinda look. (25, Mother 1, p. 56)

> I feel like screaming, 'This is my son! He has a syndrome but it's not contagious, please pay attention to him!' and I don't mean 24 hours of atten-

tion, a five-minute or a five-second 'How are you getting on?' ... that. (. . .) I'm feeling awful, they ignore me . . . I will **not** be ignored. (6, p. 9, 44)

A more general theme that was developed from parents' accounts of their dissatisfaction with some nurses' approaches was their criticism of nurses' professional detachment. Parents spoke of this as though it were synonymous with aloofness and indicative of a lack of caring which created a perceptible 'gap' between themselves and the nurses. As one mother observed:

There's such a wall there . . . there seems to be a wall that's awfully hard to get through and it's not just personalities. (6, p. 10)

Another mother spoke of this when I asked if her relationship with the nurses had altered during her stay: 'No . . . with a few, maybe . . . but mainly it's sort of . . . there's a gap' (4, p. 19). The parents seemed to have a different and far less positive view of the concept of professionalism from that commonly found in nursing literature:

Some of them have a slightly . . . you feel, a bit aloof in a way. They present a sort of front. . . . The ones that you can't speak to easier are the ones who are very sort of . . . present a very super-efficient air. (. . .) The girl who is pregnant is very, very nice, but the other one was quite . . . kind of brisk, and very . . . . . . She was being very professional in her approach. (9, p. 25)

Other parents described nurses' approaches as being professional, meaning that some nurses were detached and almost indifferent to their emotional needs. One parent described how she had been so upset by her child's injuries and subsequent treatments that it had been arranged for her to be 'sent to see a social worker'. When I asked if a nurse could have fulfilled this role she explained that she believed that such concerned attention was incompatible with the 'professional' approach:

No, they're not the same. (. . .) It's the more professional thing. (. . .) I don't think they [the nurses] are meant to be affectionate towards folk. I think they're just meant to get on with the job and do it, do their job and that's it. (25, Mother 2, p. 26, 28)

Several parents described how they viewed some nurses as being 'young girls' or 'just wee lassies'. This was not only a concern about nurses' youth, but that, as young women who did not have children of their own, they could not reasonably be expected to have a sense of empathy with the mothers.

I think because you're a parent, you see these sort of things [crying babies] and because I'm a parent I would go over and see what was wrong, but because so many of them [the nurses] are young and don't have kids . . . maybe there's no maternal instinct, or not the same amount. (28, Mother 2, p. 9)

> Half the time I don't think they knew what they were doing really . . . they hadn't sort of . . . I don't know really . . . they just . . . they looked like sort of youngsters coming from school. (2, p. 6–7)

> A lot of nurses up there are only young lassies and they've not got a family of their own and they don't realize what it's like. (25, Mother 1, p. 19)

This combination of youth and perceived inexperience could shake a parent's confidence. Another mother described, almost in a rage during the interview, how she had stood with her husband in the treatment room while two student nurses had fumblingly performed a dressing change on her six-and-a-half-month-old baby:

> My husband and I were out in a cold sweat watching a junior nurse doing our child's dressing. (. . .) This wee girl had been doing them. (. . .) The sweat used to pour off him 'cos it was so painful. . . . There was two young girls, you know them, just wee school lassies really, and the one that was doing the dressing said to this wee girl, 'You have done dressings before, haven't you?' and she said, 'Well, we had a talk about it.' (. . .) I was about passing out listening to my child crying, she didn't have a **clue**. (26, Mother 5, p. 46–47)

For some parents their isolation was heightened when they felt that they were being cared for by nurses who did not truly understand their situation. They felt no common sense of parenthood with these nurses at a time when being a parent had taken on its most primordial importance. The general impression gained from parents was that they felt that both they and their child received a qualitatively poorer standard of care from a nurse who was not herself a mother. Parents felt that nurses who had children of their own were more likely to have the experience and understanding necessary to better appreciate the situation of the live-in parents. As these parents explained:

> A few nurses have said to me that they feel differently now that they have had their own children than they used to before they had their own child, and it's one thing to nurse children who are other people's . . . (. . .) so I think, unless nurses have been in that situation, I don't think they can really understand it. (26, Mother 1, p. 109)

> You know the difference when you've got a nurse in with you that's got kids of her own and you know when you've got a nurse that's no got kids of her own (. . .) it's just their whole manner (. . .) the way they treat the children and everything. (25, Mother 1, p. 79)

This was an understanding echoed by some nurses who had returned to practice after having children. These nurses described how they viewed paediatric nursing and live-in parents markedly differently now that they were parents themselves. For these nurses, this change had not come about through professional education or practice. The change was more ontological than epistemological. Their way of being-in-the-world had altered fundamentally (Bergum, 1988; Van Manen, 1990). They were now parents and the horizon of their concerns had shifted markedly, an idea supported by recent studies of parenthood within differing contexts (Park, 1991; Leonard, 1991).

The negative experiences that parents described in their interactions with nurses were very similar to those described by Drew (1986), who carried out a phenomenological investigation of patients' experiences of exclusion and confirmation with their caregivers. Drew found that, for patients, feelings of exclusion were created by caregivers who were 'lacking in emotional warmth' and who appeared to have a 'negative regard for the subject'. 'In a general sense', stated Drew, 'what the subjects described were caregivers whom they felt had not cared for them' (Drew, 1986, p. 41).

5.3 THE DEVELOPING RELATIONSHIP BETWEEN PARENTS AND NURSES

I had considered initially that nurse–parent relationships might improve over time, in that the longer a parent lived-in, the closer and more engaged their relationship with nurses would become. While this seemed to be partly supported, it would be wrong to consider the developing relationship as being simply a function of time. There were other equally important mediators of this relationship. It was significant in this respect that nurses would speak of parents who had 'been in too long'. These parents were described by nurses as having almost outlived their usefulness and now becoming more of a liability than an asset. This will be discussed more fully in the nurses' section.

The most striking aspect of this changing relationship was the way in which some parents described how successfully their relationship with nurses had developed from being a rather detached and anonymous nurse–parent relationship to one where they considered the nurses to be more like 'friends'. However, not all parents experienced such positive relationships and some described their contacts with nurses in ways that indicated that no satisfactory or satisfying relationships had developed at all.

5.3.1 Initial encounters

Several parents mentioned a special relationship with a nurse who had been present when their child had first been admitted. Parents also described a reassuring continuity when this nurse cared for their child in the future and valued someone who had been 'there from the start'. One father had a particularly good relationship with Staff Nurse 'Patricia' that he attributed to a connectedness in that they had both experienced the trauma of his son's admission with potentially fatal scalds:

Staff Nurse Patricia was the one that always . . . I think it was the connection we got when she approached me out there [when father was waiting in the corridor outside the ICU], and I always felt . . . that . . . you know, where doctors wouldn't tell me . . . (18, p. 54)

Another mother felt that her relationship with a staff nurse had been positively influenced by the fact that the nurse had cared for her child when she had been first admitted. She described their relationship as:

Great . . . really great . . . 'cos Vera was on the first day we came in, she was there the first day and she's been great. (15, p. 21)

Another mother described a similar connectedness with nurses who had helped to care for her baby when he had been first admitted, during what she called his 'black days'. These nurses had stood within her world and concerns, they had shared this very difficult time and so they knew the person of her baby as opposed to other nurses who might have been equally competent but still lacked this vital insight.

There are others who are good nurses but who don't know him and he's just another patient to them and they haven't seen him through the black days . . . the days when he was really, really sick. (17, p. 22)

In contrast, when parents' first impressions of nurses were negative it was unlikely that they would change. No parent who was interviewed described a situation where they had 'got off to a bad start' with a nurse and later developed a good relationship. This mother's comments were typical in this respect:

Well, with the ones [the nurses] who are indifferent, I stay indifferent, I don't change my relationship with them. (6, p. 33–34)

In Chapter 2 I showed that nurses tended to 'assess' parents on first impressions. Similarly, nurses seemed to be judged by parents on first impressions. If these were not good, this damaged future chances of developing a more positive relationship. A salient feature here was that the live-in parents were in a far from normal situation and, consequently, did not behave in what they considered to be 'normal' ways. At a time when parents' emotions and anxieties were heightened, they were also more likely to be sensitive to nurses' perceived indifference or rudeness and to direct their own anger and frustrations towards nurses. This mother explained these feelings also.

There are times when you think, why me? and you get really angry and go out and kick the car or . . . anybody that's standing there (laughs) or you bite somebody's head off, you're rude, you're irritable, just everything that you would expect in a situation like that. . . . Your emotions are up and down, you're in turmoil, basically. (17, p. 19–20)

At such times an added onus was placed upon nurses to establish a good relationship from their earliest contact with parents, for such good first impressions can form the basis of a relationship that can improve and develop.

5.3.2 From professional and parent to 'a special relationship'

Parents described the nurses that they valued most almost entirely in terms of their caring qualities rather than their technical skills. Nurses who remained detached and professional in their approach were seen as being virtually uninterested and certainly as being of little help to parents. This contrasted with parents' descriptions of valued relationships that were more like friendships:

> **Father:** A lot of the nurses . . . we've been in that long, it's as if they're just pals, know what I mean?
> **Mother:** A special relationship.
> **Father:** Aye, it's not a nurse . . . a nurse–patient or a nurse–parent . . . you know, it seems to develop into **us**, I mean you can talk as if it's someone you've known for ages. (5, p. 5–6)

> I would reckon that we've made a lot of good friends with the nurses in here. (27, Mother 4, p. 51)

> I find it quite easy [talking to nurses about her emotions and feelings] because I feel that they understand . . . well certain nurses again . . . it's not just nurses full stop . . . it's nurses that I would say have become friends, that I feel I can talk to them about it, but they're the only ones. (17, p. 56)

> They [the nurses] were always friendly, but it's grown into a relationship now . . . that's my view anyway . . . I don't know how they feel (laughs) . . . but really they have become friends . . . in a way – this sounds absolutely amazing, but when I was at home I missed them! (17, p. 79)

The contrast here was dramatic between parents who described relationships of engagement, mutuality and openness with nurses as people and those parents whose discourse was restricted to terms of an obligatory respect for nurses as an occupational group and for their busyness.

Parents especially valued being able to talk with nurses in a friendly way. They could chat to them about relatively unimportant and trivial matters but, equally, they could discuss with them the much more serious aspects of their feelings and concerns. This willingness of nurses to engage in everyday social conversation with parents was highly valued. Not only was this a relief for parents in 'taking their mind off things' for a short while. It was also an important way of keeping in contact with the outside world. Significantly here, parents often described their stay in hospital half-jokingly using prison metaphors. They talked of being 'in Colditz', of relatives 'bringing in food parcels', and of 'getting paroled' to go home to see their husband and other children for a day or two. They were therefore pleased to be able to chat normally about everyday matters within a relationship that was becoming more personal and connected and less clinical (Morse, 1991). As these parents explained:

> There was one night I was even talking about football, you know what I mean, we just spoke about everything, it was really good. (5, p. 11)

You find yourself chattering about other things and you just interact much more easily. (27, Mother 1, p. 52)

There's two nurses on this afternoon who've been on the rest of the week and they're great 'cos they've come up and said about . . . one's buying a flat and, you know, where they live and what they've done and that's lovely 'cos I've managed to have a chat with them, away from hospitals and illness and babies. (2, p. 27)

This last mother's account illustrated another aspect of nurses' valued caring practices. When nurses shared biographical information about themselves in conversation with parents this seemed to enable the parents to maintain a connection with the world that they had temporarily left. It also allowed them to see the real person behind the nurse's professional front and seemed to confirm the personhood of the parent. One mother explained this clearly:

PD: What kind of things might they [nurses] do where you would think, gosh, they're treating me as a person. . . ?
Mother: I suppose when they start talking about things other than your kid and how you got here . . . talking about more personal things . . . start talking about what they did the night before or what they plan doing tonight or . . . (13, p. 30)

These parents' accounts of their developing relationships with nurses revealed the central importance of nurses' caring, involved stance in the situation. As one mother explained, these nurses were 'the only ones' that she could talk to. I suggest that this was not merely because the nurse happened to be there for a longer period of time than any other health-care professional. Rather, the nurses that were valued and that parents related to had cared sufficiently to transcend the traditional, more detached view of the nurse–parent relationship with the degree of involvement and engagement in the situation that this implies. The value of such an involvement for both nurses and patients has been proposed by Gadow (1980; 1985) who advances this idea as part of her concept of existential advocacy. Gadow (1980) argues that 'regarding the patient as a "whole" requires nothing less than the nurse acting as a "whole" person therefore the nurse who withholds parts of the self is unlikely to allow the patient to emerge as a whole' (Gadow, 1980, p. 87) and that 'professional involvement is not an alternative to other kinds of involvement, such as emotional, aesthetic, physical, or intellectual. It is a deliberate synthesis of all of these, a participation of the entire self, using every dimension of the person as a resource in the professional relation' (Gadow, 1980, p. 90).

Nurses who were described so positively had taken a truly holistic view of parents and recognized them as being both individuals and members of families, rather than as merely an extension of their child's illness or the objects upon which nurses practised paediatric nursing. They responded not with detached professional selves but with their concerned human selves, thus allowing parents to show up as persons who needed to give and receive care.

Parents' descriptions of their evolving relationships with nurses suggested that their length of stay was important, in that the longer they lived-in, the more opportunities they had to get to know nurses. However, linear time to the parents was of secondary importance to the nurses' caring way of being (Roach, 1987; Benner, 1988). Nurses, through their caring practices, helped parents to establish and develop a satisfying relationship. They created time to be with the parents and child that confirmed the parent's own sense of worth and value.

5.4 NURSES' RELATIONSHIPS WITH LIVE-IN PARENTS

Social phenomena such as the relationships between nurses and live-in parents are co-created rather than unilateral. In this section I examine the relationships that developed between parents and nurses from the nurses' perspective. Relationships are recognized as being elusive concepts to describe and explain but they are equally well recognized as being of central importance within nursing. One way of trying to uncover relationships is to examine the ways in which they are made visible. This is approached through an exploration of the nurses' understandings of their work and of how nurses' practices revealed their working out of ideas of parents and families.

5.4.1 Creating the relationship: connecting with parents

The nurses' narratives described how they tried to establish a relationship with live-in parents that allowed both of them to function in what nurses saw as their different and respective roles. A common feature of the nurses' accounts was that they often qualified their responses by saying that their approaches to, or feelings regarding parents would 'depend on the parents' or 'vary between parents'. These nurses found it difficult to give generalized responses to questions and would therefore use stories of a particular parent or family to illustrate a particular approach. One nurse explained how this ability to consider parents as individuals had become so embedded within her everyday practices, that it was difficult to recognize, even upon reflection:

> I'm more aware that now I actually change myself depending on the parents. I don't think ... I sometimes am aware afterwards that I've come across almost as ... almost as this nice staff nurse in the white dress that's giving them a straightforward view, and other times I'm more friendly ... ... not friendly, more relaxed with them and giving them more.... I do have a different attitude depending on the parents (. . .) I don't look at them and say, 'I'm going to put this or that hat on for this person.' I'm only aware sometimes afterwards of how I've changed. (7, p. 37–38)

Treating parents as unique persons and differentiating between their perceived needs was used by some nurses as a way to help them connect with the particular person of each parent. In the same way, they explained that each child was unique and that they too required such an individual approach. However, such an approach was constrained within the context of the ward. The nurses often articulated an individualistic philosophy regarding parents, but it was clear from the accounts of some parents that such a belief in individual approaches was, by itself, unable to create within the parents the feeling that their unique situation was being respected.

Nurses who were concerned for parents as persons were aware of the tensions and difficulties inherent in trying to accommodate such a perspective within the ward. The essence of this tension was the problem of trying to reconcile the needs and wishes of individual parents and children with the often competing demands of others and of the ward and hospital as a whole.

This was a tension that could show up in the most everyday of practices. One nurse described this as she related how she had reluctantly refused a mother's request to make some toast for her son's supper. The nurse recognized that this might have seemed an innocuous and reasonable request from the mother's perspective, and indeed this was congruent with her own personal philosophy that emphasized the importance of treating each parent and child as an individual. However the nurse felt that she had to balance this reasonable request against other contextual factors. She argued that she had been particularly busy at this point in the evening and could not have justifiably 'dropped everything' to go and make toast. The nurse explained that

> The night sisters had said that mums weren't allowed in the kitchen, even to make toast, but that isn't why I did it [refused permission]. We were quite busy and I didn't have time and nobody else had time to go and make toast and she said, 'Oh I'll make it for him.' But I said, 'Yeah, but not all of the mums are in to make toast for all of the kids and I can't have you making it for them all.' (. . .) I was nice about it but I felt bad. (32, p. 24)

The nurse also felt that such an action could have established a precedent with possible consequences with which she could not have coped, namely, that any number of other parents in the ward might consequently have made a similar request that she could not then have legitimately refused. The nurse did not take this decision lightly. She expressed a profound concern that such tensions between the individual expectations of the parents and the more universal concerns of the nurses had a detrimental impact on the nurse–parent relationship. As she explained:

> It's hard to cope with, 'cos you don't want to be a baddie, you know, you've known them a while, you've built up a good relationship with them and you don't want to sound the baddie by saying no, but sometimes you get put in a position where you say, 'What do I do here?' . . . and it's very hard to . . . . . . to show some authority when you're really friendly with the parents, you know. . . . (32, p. 27)

This nurse's account revealed the tensions that she experienced as she tried to reconcile the wishes of an individual parent with the universal concerns of the ward. This account highlighted a neglected area within the nurse–parent relationship that has a mirror image in the literature concerning nurses and patients. The literature on nurse–patient relationships has tended to suggest that such relationships are polar opposites where nurses will either practise 'individual patient care' or batch-treat people as social or medical 'types'. Davis (1984) exemplifies this view: 'Although the trend over the past few years has been towards the individualized, planned and documented care of the nursing process, there is much evidence to suggest that, then as well as now, nurses tend to deal with types of people, types of behaviour and types of disease, rather than individuals' (Davis, 1984, p. 70).

Attempts to characterize the nurse–parent relationship in this way as being either–or with respect to the individual versus collective are, I suggest, mistaken. Such a simplistic concept ignores the complexity of clinical practice where nurses do not make a free, ideological choice between two abstract polarities. Learning the skills of involvement with parents is an infinitely more complex part of skilled nursing practice than typologies can accommodate (Benner, 1990c; Morse, 1991).

5.4.2 Initial encounters and intuitive assessments

The nurses' accounts of their relationships with parents revealed a belief that the quality of the developing relationships was largely dependent upon the parents themselves. The nurses generally shared a perception of the fixed nature of a parent's personality. They believed that the initial period of hospitalization was important for future relationships. During this initial period, the nurses took their cues as to what kind of parent and person they were dealing with and consequently determined how the nurse–parent relationship was likely to develop. As one nurse observed:

> You can suss out almost immediately the ones that are ... the ones that aren't there all day but are caring and the ones that aren't there all day 'cos they can't be bothered. (16, p. 53)

Nurses described the parent's personality as being vital for the formation of good relationships. They frequently stressed the parental side of the relationship equation, but seemed less aware that their approach was influential. A nurse in a focus group interview contradicted her colleague on this point:

> **Nurse C:** Definitely the attitudes of the parents and their personality.
> **Nurse A:** I would say the attitudes of parents **and** nurses, I don't think you can just say parents. ... (31, p. 24)

Personality was used generically by nurses to describe the behaviours and attitudes that they would assess in parents as they formulated their important first impressions. Not surprisingly, the parental characteristics that they rated positively included friendliness, gratefulness, responsiveness and an expressed caring concern for the child. Conversely, unfavourable displays of parents' personality included aggressiveness, excessive questioning, non -responsiveness, being excessively demanding and failing to show care or concern for the child.

The nurses spoke of the beginnings of their relationship with parents in ways which suggested that their first impressions of parents were powerful influences upon the subsequent relationship. First impressions could almost make or break potential relationships. One nurse conveyed this immediacy well when she spoke of 'hitting it off' with parents:

> I feel it's like a lot of situations where – you could compare it with a social situation where if you just happen to hit it off with the people then it makes a good relationship; it's like anything else, you just meet the parents and you might hit it off with them . . . or you meet parents that you don't hit it off with. (20, p. 51)

Nurses described other ways in which first impressions were important in setting the groundwork upon which future relationships might develop. For example, nurses claimed to be able to tell almost immediately the extent of involvement that parents might wish to have:

> You can sort of see initially whether, you know, they want to be there but don't really want to do much with them. (7, p. 7)

> **Nurse A:** I suppose it's first impressions as well, working in any sort of situation, 'cos recently we had a dad and the first thing he asked me about was . . . about filling out his form for bus fares, not how his child was, the first question was, 'How do I claim this?' . . . (laughs) . . . now that kinda put my back up, I must admit.. . .
> **Nurse C:** But you do, you make judgements on your initial . . .
> **Nurse A:** . . . so I suppose first impressions mean a lot. (31, p. 25–26)

For the nurse–parent relationship to develop, it was important for parents to 'come to terms with' their situation and the implications of their child's illness or injury. The presence or extent of this parental acceptance was another aspect which nurses felt able to ascertain almost immediately.

> It's like your initial – it's the way they react to the initial injury that makes you think, right, they've accepted this and this is how we go on from here. (30, p. 9)

The most formal initial encounter between parents and nurses was the child's admission. Nurses described this as being an important event in the formation of their initial impressions of parents, especially in relation to assessing their 'problems' and the degree of involvement that they might appear to wish for.

> When you're admitting the child and doing his profile is usually quite a good time to assess how much they know and what they want to know and

how involved they want to be and any other problems that are going to stop them being involved. (11, p. 10–11)

I think if you've been involved with that child's admission, your rapport with that set of parents is completely different. (. . .) I've always felt that I know the parents more if I've admitted their child. (19, p. 36)

I argue that nurses' repeated references to parents' personalities cannot be adequately interpreted from a strictly psychological perspective that views personality as being essentially internal and fixed. The prominence of parents' personality as an explanatory factor could advance or retreat depending upon, for example the success of the child's treatment or of nursing interventions. Where nurse–parent relationships had not developed positively or were overtly hostile, the parent's personality loomed large. It was common in many nurses' accounts for them to absolve themselves from all responsibility for this situation by claiming that there was nothing that they could do about the problem relationship as this was just the type of person that the parent was. Where nurse–parent relationships were more positive and mutually satisfying, personality would be eclipsed as an explanation by other factors, the most frequently mentioned being the greater length of the parent's stay, their becoming more relaxed and 'settling in', their increasing familiarity with the ward, staff and routines, or simply that their child was getting better and thus they were much less anxious. As these nurses noted:

I think that they become more familiar with the nurses and I think that they become part of the ward. (. . .) I think the mums become more settled (. . .) and I think that the rapport gets better. (16, p. 67)

I think also it depends whether it's a long- or a short-stay parent (. . .) like, some of our parents have been in for a long, long time and we have a super relationship. (29, Nurse C, p. 10)

Nurses commented that their initial impressions of parents were constructed in exactly the same way that they would form initial impressions of other people in their everyday social lives. As one nurse noted, 'we can't help doing it, we're only human'. In this respect, it would be reasonable to assume that the relationship between nurses and parents might improve over the duration of the parents' stay. This too, however, was a more complex facet of the nurse–parent relationship than was originally imagined.

5.4.3 Having sustained contact with parents

The nurses relied considerably upon their first impressions of what they referred to as the parent's personality in the formation of their initial relationships with parents. However, the nurse–parent relationship was not static and developed over time while simultaneously being shaped by other factors.

The nature of the child's illness or injury influenced the development of the nurse–parent relationship in several ways. First, nurses explained that when children and their parents were admitted for 'minor' reasons, where the child was not seriously ill, there was less likelihood of a close relationship with the parents developing. This was because the nurses believed that most of their attention was necessarily devoted to the more seriously ill and demanding children. As one nurse explained during a focus group:

> I think the iller the child is, the more support the parents get, which is OK ... fine ... if you've got a very sick child they need a lot of support but you forget the kid that fell over and banged his head, I mean that may be just as traumatic to the parents as what somebody that's having a major by-pass is [sic] and those are the parents that tend to get 'Oh the mother's unit's down there', and 'Get a cup of tea downstairs' (makes a dismissive gesture with her hand) and nobody really bothers with them 'cos they're only going to be in for one night. . . . (29, p. 54)

This nurse described a common influence on the nurse–parent relationship, the parent's length of stay. There was general agreement among the nurses that relationships with parents were qualitatively better the longer the parents were living-in but further exploration of this point revealed that this was not a purely chronological phenomenon.

Other equally important influences were at work. Nurses felt that they had little or no relationship with parents who only stayed with their child during a short admission, perhaps for observation following a head injury or febrile convulsion, or whose child was undergoing day or overnight surgery. A nurse explained that

> Kids that are in overnight or two nights, I mean they [the parents] don't make much effort to have contact with us when it's not needed, it's just when are they getting home and what do they have to do when they get home, that's all. (11, p. 27)

This nurse shared a common belief with her colleagues that the determinants of the nurse–parent relationship were located within the parent. It was they who did not make the effort that was assumed to be largely their responsibility. Nurses felt that parents became more involved in their child's care as their stay progressed. One nurse described this:

> I think probably the length of time they've been in . . . . I mean, you wouldn't instantly expect a child that comes in very ill, being tube-fed, for the mum to instantly tube-feed the child, but after they've been in for a week, two weeks and things are stable then you start expecting the parents to participate in care. (3, p. 4)

Previous discussions of nurses' perceptions of parents suggested that, for nurses, a successful relationship would have to be premised upon parents being willing and eager to participate, particularly in the basic mothering work. The nurses explained how the quality of their relationship with parents could improve with the length of parent's stay. Nurses spoke of becoming more friendly with parents, of discovering more about their personal and family lives and of the communication between the two groups improving due to the coming down of barriers between nurse and parent. Nurses described this change:

> The longer that they're in then the more you're able to almost have a joke, even with a child who's been ill for a while, sort of get a more relaxed relationship (. . .) and you seem to get a more friendly relationship with the person, you know, you get to know them and their family involvement, you don't just know the one parent, the one who's staying in, you get to know more about their family situation. (7, p. 27–28)

> I would say yes, certainly, parents who have been in for a long time, you do become really friendly with them. (24, p. 20)

> I think that they become more familiar with the nurses and I think that they become part of the ward (. . .). I think that the mums become more settled, they find it easier to ask questions (. . .) and I think that the rapport gets better. (16, p. 67)

These nurses described several of the factors that mediated this change in relationship, which I characterize as progressing from a primarily impersonal and professional (in the sense used by parents) relationship to what one parent described as a 'special relationship'. This was more of a friendship that developed between parent and nurse. The nurses' descriptions of how their relationships with parents improved and progressed suggested the importance of a developing appreciation of the unique personhood of the parent, not only as an individual but within the wider context of their family relationships.

Evidence for this suggestion has already been advanced in Chapter 3 in the discussion of the case of baby 'Sasha' and the nurses' interactions with her mother. Further support for what is an important finding comes from the account of another nurse in the burns and plastic surgery ward. In Chapter 3, there is a detailed discussion of one nurse's lengthy and often highly critical account of a mother's stay. There was another nurse in the ward at this time, however, who was allocated to be something of a primary nurse for this mother. Her account of her relationship with this mother stands in contrast to the previous nurse's, marked especially by a deeper and more empathic understanding of this mother's particular problems. This nurse observed that

> I think in this mother's way, she had **so many** social problems . . . that she was trying to sort them out (. . .). She didn't feel confident enough to come and say to any of us about the problems she was having at home, and I think that a lot of it stemmed from that her husband came in here and beat her up in the corridor . . . and then the case conference about the way she

was treating her child, there was a lot of grievances aired there. (24, p. 24–25)

This nurse also described how she had come to take a different view of this mother from some of the other staff. She explained that

To me she was totally different: I didn't have as many problems with her as the rest of the staff did (. . .). I think it's 'cos I always made an effort with her . . . and I always made a point of going and speaking to her when she came into the ward. (24, p. 26)

Through taking the time and making the effort to get to know the person behind the 'social problem', this nurse came to a more empathic understanding of the lived experience of this mother as she spent an increasingly lengthy period of time as a live-in parent. The nurse noted that

It's a hard life being here all week, every day of the week, for the number of weeks that she was here . . . and thinking, there is a problem here . . . there isn't a life for them in the Mother's Unit and I think that the mothers judge each other up in the Unit . . . and I think the other thing is that there's a bit of a clique between mothers that she never really fitted in. She had a few friends when [her child] was first admitted and she kept in touch with them and that was who she used to go out with. She never really made any friends after they left and I think she was really lonely up there. (24, p. 27–28)

This nurse's narrative was conspicuously lacking in the language of control, coercion, and judgement that characterized other nurses' accounts of this mother's stay. Instead we hear a discourse of empowerment, empathy, affirmation, understanding and opening possibilities. Only when this nurse had established such connectedness and sense of knowing the person of the parent could she, for example, use humour tactfully enough to lighten tense situations or raise sensitive areas of a child's care for dialogue rather than confrontation.

5.4.4 Parents who were 'in too long'

Several nurses raised the issue of the parent who had 'been in too long'. The phrase 'parents who have been in too long' alerted me to the possibility that, while relationships might well have improved and developed over time, they might have reached a sense of 'peak', after which they might have altered or even deteriorated. Here, one nurse observed:

I think it depends: sometimes the longer parents are in, the worse they get . . . and you think, oh, these parents just need to get home . . . you know . . . they've had enough . . . they don't want to be here any longer. (29, Nurse A, p. 56)

How nurses came to perceive parents as having been 'in too long' and the effects of this upon relationships were illustrated in the following account:

PD: What would make you think that a person had been in too long?

Nurse: Just the kinda . . . lethargic mum who, instead of asking questions and being interested, just sits there . . . and being totally peed off with the whole business, and was . . . maybe feeling that she hadn't been told enough . . . even getting to the stage of being fed up, and saying, 'What's happening, is he getting home this week?'. Like, for example – can't remember his name . . . mum was living in the hostel –wee hypospadias from Dumfries . . . 'cos she was at the stage of . . . see, she was by his bedside **all the time** and she was totally burnt out by the thing . . . just an unnatural situation (. . .) and just that, sort of, burnt out and just looking for problems type of thing . . . they've been in here too long.

PD: Could you put a time limit on it?

Nurse: Two weeks . . . any more than that and they start to get fed up, especially if she has to be there most of the time, or wants to be there most of the time or thinks it's her duty to be there most of the time (. . .). I would say two to three weeks at the most, any more than that and then you start to get a weary mum or dad. (16, p. 69–71)

This account suggests that the parent who had been 'in too long' had possibly become a lingering reminder of the hospital's failure to effectively deal with the child's particular problem and return them home. Such parents became frustrated and angry at the apparent failure of the system and staff to 'do something' about their child. This sense of frustration seemed more marked where children were not receiving frequent, highly visible medical treatment or nursing care. For example, feelings of frustration with the hospital's perceived lack of therapeutic activity were expressed by the parents of the comatose children who were recovering from severe head injury, by parents of some children in the burns unit whose grafts were taking longer than expected to 'take' and by mothers whose children had been admitted for diagnostic investigations. These parents posed problems for the nurses when they consequently approached with repeated questions that a nurse felt able to respond to only by 'saying the same things again and again' (31, Nurse C, p. 31). As the above account indicated, it was also the nurse who was most likely to be the recipient of any parental anger or frustration.

The above nurse's description seemed contradictory in that both the parent's unwillingness to ask questions and show interest and their questioning regarding discharge could both be seen as indications that the parent has been 'in too long'. However, I suggest that this may be better understood in relation to the type of questions that parents who were thought to have been 'in too long' were likely to ask. These were unlikely to be the type of questions that the nurses would take as being an indication of the parent showing an interest and that the nurses would have little difficulty in responding to. From the nurses' accounts it seemed that these parents' questions were more likely to be questions that nurses felt unable to answer. This may have been because no precisely predictive answer regarding the child's future could be honestly given. In the case of the parents who asked about their child's future management or discharge date, this was information traditionally and currently considered to be the preserve of medical staff to give out.

In addition to nurse-perceived problems, parents who had been 'in too long' provided a tangible reminder to nurses of the reality of long-term chronic illness, disability and uncertainty. In an acute paediatric hospital, it has been argued, nursing and medical staff operate within a health-care perspective that emphasizes cure, repair and the dominance of medical knowledge (Robinson, 1987; Thorne and Robertson, 1988b; Knafl et al., 1988; Beuf, 1989). Parents who had been 'in too long' became a manifestation of the failure of the 'technocure' model (Benner, 1985b), of the possibility of chronic problems and of the increasing development of parental expertise and knowledge. Such parents could not be accommodated within a narrow curative perspective. Their presence forced some nurses to define them as a problem and their leaving the ward as the solution. Alternatively, and more positively, they may have been the stimulus that helped nurses to consider other perspectives of paediatric nurse caring which could better meet their needs.

5.5 PARENTS' OTHER LIVES: FAMILIES AND HOMES

Parents' and nurses' accounts suggested that the general focus of care was the sick child. As one mother noted:

> I think you feel that you're not here to be nursed, it's a children's ward, it's your child that's here to be nursed. (26, Mother 5, p. 94)

Peripheral to the child focus were the needs and concerns of the child's parents. On a farther periphery of concern were the rest of the parents' network of home, family and friends. The parents described how they received support from husbands and other relatives and friends but, significantly, they also revealed that family relationships during this time could be a source of strain.

5.5.1 The support of family and friends

The most common pattern of parental living-in was for the mother to stay in hospital with the child while the father looked after any other children at home. This might involve the father negotiating leave from work or, as in one case, of giving up his job when leave was not granted. Grandparents and other close relatives also formed part of a helping network who looked after other children, bought shopping and otherwise kept the home going in the mother's absence. It was not only such organizational and practical support that parents valued but the emotional support that families could also give.

A father described how his father-in-law had shared in his vigil while his child was in one of the intensive care areas following a serious accident. There was no accommodation available for the child's grandfather and consequently he had slept for several days in his car outside the hospital. The grandfather was particularly helpful to this family and shared the vigil shifts, sitting in the corridor outside the ICU. He tried to bolster the parents' strength and sense of hope when the child's prognosis seemed poor. For example, at one point the parents had been told that there was a possibility that their child might have suffered some brain damage. The father described the encouragement and support which his father-in-law had given:

> They says to my wife, 'Don't build your hopes up' (. . .) so my father-in-law says to me, 'He's **not** got brain damage, his eyes is not right back, he's just had a hard day in theatre' (. . .) so they said he was going on a brain scan the following day, so my father-in-law says, 'You just go home and I'll stay, but don't worry.' . . . He was a great strength, her father, he was, 'cos I'd just have went round the corner and died and that would have been me, but he was saying, 'It's all right, he's going to be all right, that wee boy's not came a week and going to give up [hasn't survived a week only to give up now].' . . . so he says, 'You go home and I'll phone you tonight,' so he phoned later at night and told us he [the child] was having a good sleep. (18, p. 26–27)

5.5.2 Maintaining home and family connections

Although parents decided to live in with their child, they could not entirely cut themselves off from their homes and families, even for a short period. Maintaining contact with their 'other life' was, however, difficult and was most frequently expressed by parents when they spoke of how they felt it 'impossible to be in two places at once'. Something had to give.

Parents usually tried to arrange to spend a night at home, perhaps once a week, in order to be with their other children or to get away from the hospital for a short while. However, many parents reported that such breaks, like meals and coffee breaks, often did not allow them to rest or 're-charge their batteries'. In some cases breaks proved to be sources of stress in themselves as parents found that they could not forget about their child in the hospital, or were short-tempered with their other children. One mother described how she had tried to go back to work for a few hours each day but found herself unable to concentrate upon anything but her child:

> I went into work this morning and I lasted till about midday and they said, 'For Christ's sake go away!' (laughs) . . . I'm shuffling all this paper about . . . no good to anybody . . . signed a few cheques and that was it. (27, Mother 4, p. 27)

Similarly, a mother tried to take a break to do the family's shopping:

> It was as much as I could do yesterday to rush out, it wasn't even as if I left him on his own, my husband came in, I rushed out, went to Safeway, got the shopping, put it away . . . and I was halfway round that supermarket and I couldn't concentrate on shopping or anything, I was pathetic. . . . (27, Mother 1, p. 27–28)

This conflict centred on 'wanting to be in two places at once' was very real for parents who on the one hand felt strongly that they wanted to live-in for their child yet at the same time missed their home and family life:

> I can't remember what it's like [her home and family life]. We went home for the night last weekend and I found I was wandering round my home looking for the other people, it seemed so strange to be on my own again, in my own house, with my own things (. . .). I suppose I'll get back to normal life again, but I can't . . . I can't remember . . . I do miss my home a lot. . . . (17, p. 50–51)

This mother had no other children, yet missed 'what a normal day was like'. Other parents missed their other children at home and tried to minimize any disruption to their lives. A desire to normalize the period of hospitalization for them characterized many of the parents' plans. Although their mother was in hospital with their brother or sister, the lives of the other children were to be kept as normal as possible. This was felt to be especially important where the other children were very young and in danger of losing their hard-won routine, perhaps by having to travel to and from the hospital with their father at unfamiliar times.

The lives of older children at home were also affected as they were expected to be better behaved, more helpful and more understanding than usual for the sake of their parents. A father described how his expectations of his other children were greater at this time of crisis:

> The oldest one realizes what's happened. I try to explain to him that he's got to try to help his daddy 'cos his daddy's got to go and see his wee brother (. . .) and if we're at home and he does something I'll say, 'Do you not think we've got enough trouble on our plate?' and he'll realize and he'll go and tidy his room up. (18, p. 47)

This father's account suggested that parents' tempers were shorter than normal at this time and that the other members of the family were liable to bear the consequences of this. Several other parents described this:

> You've got to sort of make your patience go longer [in the ward], and you find that when you go home you blow. Not literally a big massive argument, but you go home and something tiny will niggle you and you'll blow because of it. (. . .) It was about 10 days after John's accident . . . we had

not said anything wrong to each other. Nothing. Then, suddenly my husband hit my wee boy, he's eight, I think he was hitting his sister . . . and he just gave him a smack and the whole thing just **completely blew** . . . and then after we calmed down. But it had to snap, the air was too tight. You'll find yourself snapping more at home with the other children. (. . .) You come here and you're calm, or you try to be calm, you go home and the same thing happens again. You're not taking it out on the children as such, but I suppose they do suffer because you haven't got as much patience because you've used it all up. (4, p. 26–27)

Parents in one focus group interview echoed these sentiments when I asked about the effect that their living-in had on their homes and families:

Mother 1: [discussing her five-year-old daughter at home] She's struggling for a bit more attention, although she's got her dad's full attention (. . .) she's just finding it a wee bit hard to handle and you worry about your relationship with the ones that you're not seeing so often and you struggle to see them for some time each day or whatever, and then end up fighting with them (laughs) because the both of you are so uptight that. . .

Mother 2: That's the other thing, you don't want to shout at them 'cos you're not seeing them that much. . . .

Mother 4: I think you realize how tense you are, though, when you're actually with the other ones. . . .

Mother 3: You do. . . .

Mother 4: Your level of tolerance just goes absolutely downhill. (27, p. 65–66)

The dilemma of wanting to be in two places at once was very difficult for parents to deal with. While most parents made efforts to spend at least a short while at home during their stay, others found even such a short parting from their hospitalized child to be too unsettling. It seemed that, for some parents, the only way in which they could devote the exclusive energy and attention that they felt their child required, was to temporarily 'blank out' the needs of their other children. In this respect, some families were fortunate in that the father was able and willing to take on this role in his wife's absence. While this was clearly an uncomfortable choice for some mothers to make, they felt more reassured in their belief that this time offered their husbands and sons time together.

Such families, where the father was very supportive both emotionally and practically, emphasized the exceptional difficulties that faced a single parent who also had other children at home. For example, one single mother had to make her own 'Sophie's Choice' about which of her young children was most important and then try to arrange for her mother to look after the other child at home. She explained that

I want to be there every day, even though I've got the wee one at home, I'd rather be here . . . he's sort of more important. (15, p. 2)

5.5.3 Coping with the demands of families and friends

While family and friends were often supportive, a tension existed for parents regarding the nature of their contact with them. This was revealed in the accounts of parents who described how they felt obliged to manage the flow of information to their families in order to spare them any distress. They also described how they felt a need to appear as optimistic and cheerful as possible for similar reasons.

The resolution of such tensions involved more than superficial 'impression management' where parents were exclusively concerned with their public face. Parents attempted to protect themselves from what they described as an emotional and physical draining. The 'draining' metaphor conveyed that parents saw their ability to cope as finite and thus they sought ways of conserving these energies for their own use. Parents therefore felt it necessary to be less than open at times with information given to families. They also wanted to simply be alone at times rather than to be among friends.

A mother described how keeping in frequent contact with her parents had become an additional strain:

> It's getting harder now as time goes on, although Jamie's getting better and better. . . . I'm finding it really . . . it's draining and I find that I don't want to phone my mother now because I don't want to have to . . . sound all . . . (gestures with a smile indicating cheerful and optimistic). (17, p. 52–53)

Other parents in a focus group discussion explained that there were times when the attentions of families and friends were an additional source of stress rather that a welcome concern, despite their kindly intentions:

> **Mother 2:** You're going home and the phone's ringing and folk are coming to the door and you're saying, 'Look, I'll talk to you later, I have to get back to the hospital' and you think, what did I come home for? . . . You make a cup of tea and you don't get the chance to drink it, you're so busy.
> **Mother 1:** I don't know about you, but if you see people coming to the door and the phone's ringing . . . I find it really difficult. . . . I mean, Brian's only been in a few days and he's still quite ill and I don't really **want** to talk to everybody about it. . . . I mean, I know the family are all concerned but I'd rather they talked to somebody else, you know?
> **Mother 2:** I say this to my husband. . . . He got home last night and two neighbours came to the door and the phone was ringing . . . he just says to people, 'She's stable', but you have to be . . . if it was their child, you'd be the same. . . . It's nice that people are concerned, but it takes up a lot . . . (. . .) sort of chatting and then you say, 'God, here I am, I come home for 10 minutes' peace' and you'd be as well staying in the hospital. (27, p. 34–36)

Parents' own parents were often a source of help and support during the child's hospitalization but again a balance had to be struck regarding the extent of their involvement and the amount and nature of any information that parents felt able to disclose. Parents felt it important to inform their own parents as to the child's condition and suggested that it would be difficult to expect their help and support if parents were thought to be withholding this information. However, there were factors that mitigated against such a degree of openness which parents had to take into account. For example, would the information cause their parents undue distress? Was there any point in informing them since, as one mother remarked, 'there's not really anything that they can do'? One mother provided a poignant exemplar of how such a tension could develop:

> I'm really quite cold to my own mother, but Jill was brought in on the Saturday and my father was having open-heart surgery on the Monday, so we . . . we told mum that Jill only had a kidney infection and she needed a wee drip just to keep her going [Jill was in fact much more ill with a serious renal disorder] . . . playing it down . . . and my dad died last Saturday (. . .) so really, where my mother would have been very supportive, and I know she would have been, you couldn't tell her, you know . . . we kept saying, 'Oh she's just being a wee bit sick so they put a wee drip in . . .' (. . .) and the day that he died, you know, I had to say to mum, she really is ill and I can't leave her . . . I can't come and be with you (. . .) so it was really hard. . . . So, where I appreciate what you're saying, you don't really want to talk to a lot of people, I really could have done with my mother . . . I really could have, it was difficult. (27, Mother 4, p. 37–38)

When this mother spoke of being cold towards her own mother, it is unlikely from her comments that this implied a dislike. It seems more probable that this was another attempt by a mother to try to 'blank out' events or even people who might, through their demands upon herself and her time, have lessened the time and attention that she felt she must give to her daughter. Her dilemma was that she had to play down the severity of her daughter's illness in order to protect her mother and, indirectly, herself.

The possibility against which she had guarded, was that, if she had told her mother 'the worst', her mother might have reacted to the truth in such a way as to have required support from her daughter. This would have been a support that would have further 'drained' what the mother perceived to be her limited resources. She also recognized that her own mother faced a similar dilemma in that she had major worries of her own regarding her husband's surgery. In addition, her mother had her own grief to deal with following the death of her husband. Had this mother been completely honest about her child's condition, she believed that she would have caused her mother an additional and possibly unnecessary burden.

For most live-in parents, the help and support from their spouses, other children, family and friends was valued. This help may have been essentially practical, such as looking after other children, or more akin to emotional or social support. The nature of this support, however, was more complex than this simple categorization suggests. It cannot be assumed that family and friends were, *per se*, always supportive and valued by parents. Much depended upon how parents felt that they could deal with such people at any given time during their child's hospitalization. This relational and contextual dimension was difficult for parents, and indeed for family and friends, to acknowledge. What was effectively suggested was that there were times when the expressed concern of family and friends were valued and times when they were not. Such selective gratitude was not easy for parents to express or for others to accept.

Another important theme that emerged from the interpretation of parents' discussions of families was that their ability to 'spread themselves around', both physically and emotionally, was limited. They felt unable to devote themselves to their sick child and continue as before with their myriad of other concerns and responsibilities. Not only could they not be in two places at once, neither could they be five people at once.

Parents remarked that it was 'only natural' for people to express concern and to wish to help them at a traumatic time. However, there were times when the most valued facility would have been simply the opportunity to be alone with each other not in the sense of being ignored and neglected, but in being afforded a comfortable privacy that seemed to be unavailable. As one mother explained:

> I feel that when your baby's really sick, like ours was, you need somewhere that's really private, you can't be really private in the Mothers' Unit, you can't be really private anywhere in the hospital. (17, p. 58)

Parents expressed a desire for privacy particularly during extremely stressful or distressing moments. However, an important part of the context of the parents' lived experiences were their relationships and encounters with other live-in parents.

5.6 RELATIONSHIPS BETWEEN PARENTS: ALONE TOGETHER

My previous experience as a paediatric nurse and subsequently as a paediatric nursing teacher made me aware of a tendency in some nurses to treat the relationships that developed between parents with some suspicion. The view was often expressed by students that such 'unofficial parent groups', as I term them, did not function in anyone's best interests. Almost invariably, they were perceived as a source of uninformed gossip about children's treatments or, more seriously, as a conspiracy of criticism against the nurses and the hospital. It was unusual for nurses to acknowledge that friendships and close relationships formed among parents. Nor did I gain a sense that such relationships were perceived to be beneficial. This view was largely endorsed by what I saw and heard during the research fieldwork. Nurses were often suspicious rather than supportive of the relationships that parents formed and were more likely to speak of the problems such relationships could engender. It seemed to be the exception when nurses spoke positively of such contacts or described how they encouraged contact between parents in order that they could offer each other mutual understanding and support.

The parents' accounts suggested that the relationships that existed among parents were as complex and subtle as those that existed between parents and nurses. For example, I assumed that parents might consider that they had a common bond or purpose by virtue of the fact that they were all parents who were living-in with their sick or injured child. This was the notion that they were 'all in the same boat'. However, the fact that they were all live-in parents of a sick child was often an insufficient basis upon which to constitute any real sense of unity or shared identity. For this sense of common purpose was tempered by both parents' and staff views that all children were unique and different. No-one's child was quite the same as yours and, in this situation, not to be identical was to be significantly different.

Parents also described the difficulties that they faced in being understanding of the needs of other children and their parents while trying to act as their own child's advocate. This demanded a degree of what one mother described as 'selfishness'. They were there, as another mother explained, to 'make sure that I get the best possible care for my child'. Co-existing with these tensions, however, were accounts of mutual support and concern and many parents seemed to have found the help and support offered by other live-in parents to be valuable.

5.6.1 Parents' shared concerns and identities: 'all in the same boat'?

Although some parents spoke of feeling a common bond with other parents, others felt much more isolated in their situation. The parents in one group interview described how they experienced a connectedness with others:

> **Mother 2:** The girl I'm sharing a room with now, I don't see her all day and I've only slept with her two nights (laughs) . . . and I feel I've got to know her quite well (. . .) and I could say that I really like her. (. . .) I feel even in this short time I know her as well as somebody in my street that I only say good morning to. . . .
> **Mother 4:** And you're kind of bonded anyway, 'cos everybody's child's ill.
> **Mother 2:** Well, that's right.
> **Mother 4:** . . . so you've got that common thing between everyone. (27, p. 53–54)

From this account it might appear that parents easily formed alliances and felt a sense of shared identity with each other based solely on the fact that they were living-in with their sick child. Parents' further descriptions and explanations of their relationships suggested, however, that this is too simplistic an interpretation. There were additional factors that affected parents' relationships with other live-in parents who were ostensibly 'in the same boat'.

Many parents described how the nature and severity of their child's illness were major factors in constituting their relationship with other parents. While they may have felt a communality with other parents, they could easily feel isolated and alienated by the uniqueness or by the severity of their child's condition. The mother of a very seriously ill baby explained this particularly clearly:

> The mothers of the children with leukaemia, they stick together because (. . .) they're coming across the same problems. . . . Jamie's so peculiar . . . Jamie's problems are all of his own, nobody's like him, so . . . I've been chatting with a couple of mothers on the ward whose babies are in with bronchiolitis (. . .) of course they're quite shocked when I say that Jamie was in [another hospital] with bronchiolitis, and look at him now, you know, hanging on to his life . . . they don't like talking to me too long (laughs) . . . dear God, no . . . 'Look what happened to her baby! Get away from this woman quick!' (. . .) I can't really talk to other mums about it because they're in here with their own problems, and if they're not in here with a really bad problem . . . you . . . you don't really want to talk to somebody that's in with a kid who's got tonsillitis, although that can be serious, but you know, . . . when your baby's life's in danger. . . (17, p. 56, 69–70)

Jamie's mother articulated this dilemma particularly vividly as she described how she felt isolated due to Jamie's unique medical biography. Her sense of isolation was emphasized by her recognition that some groups of parents had formed an informal supportive network for each other. This seemed most apparent when they had the common purpose that arose from their children all having similar problems, as with the parents of children with leukaemia that she mentioned. However, even a shared diagnosis of bronchiolitis was insufficient to connect her with other mothers of babies with this fairly common paediatric illness. Jamie's precarious existence seemed to have created a contagion of horror that further inhibited his mother's ability to share her experience with other mothers. The final twist to this dilemma was that Jamie's mother found herself in a 'Catch-22' situation. She could not speak about Jamie with a mother whose child was as seriously ill, for she recognized that they 'had their own problems' that her experience had taught her were considerable. Nor could she speak to mothers whose children had comparatively trivial problems, for their experiences could have no real resonance with hers.

Other mothers expressed a common view, that no one else seemed able to really understand their particular situation, when they explained that

> There's nobody comes and says 'I've been through that, my daughter was **exactly** the same,' you know, they'll say, 'I had a niece who had an accident and she was very bad but she's fine now,' but to be very bad and exactly the same is completely different. (4, p. 12–13)

and similarly

> I think that you get quite selfish about your own child. . . . They're not all

in the same boat: your child is worse than theirs, your child is **ill** – and is their child as ill as your child? (6, p. 5)

When I asked if other parents had been a source of support the first of these mothers explained:

No, I don't think so, because nobody is in the same position as you: I mean, when I look at Kim [another child in the ward who had suffered a head injury], she's a lot worse than John. (4, p. 11)

The chance to meet other parents whose children had similar problems was valued by parents. Two parents told how such a meeting had been engineered by hospital staff who shared the view that such contacts were supportive and valuable. The two parents, whose children had both been admitted with a very rare disorder, discussed how their relationship had developed:

Mother 2: Well, because Claire's in a ward by herself, I don't really know that [very] many of the parents . . . apart from [Jill's mum] and I mean I was that grateful to meet Jill's mum because Jill was in the same condition that Claire's in and it was a great comfort, and they came and spoke to us.
Mother 4: That didn't really happen to us: I mean, Jill was admitted two weeks before Claire (. . .) and Dr Green came and asked us if we would go down and speak to Claire's parents and, yeah, of course we did, and then you came up and saw us. . . .
Mother 2: . . . and it gave us a lot of comfort, you know, 'cos Claire was, I mean she still is very ill . . . but you feel you're in a boat by yourself and nobody's ever been in this position before (. . .) and the nurse said that Jill's mum and dad said they would come down and see you, and it was great, 'cos when your husband sort of . . . my husband had a right sort of guilt complex about when we were in Spain [Claire had become ill while on holiday abroad and had been flown home by air-ambulance] we were told that we had to make her drink a lot because she was dehydrated, and she wouldn't drink and it was a case of forcing her, and then it turned out to be the wrong thing to be doing, and my husband had this real guilt complex about this and then your husband came and he knows all about it, and it's like listening to one of the doctors (laughs), and he's reeling off all of this condition and I thought, right enough, he's telling me all of what Claire's been through and it's because Jill's had it and he said that it was exactly the same, that he was forcing Jill to drink . . . and it did make us feel a whole lot better. (27, p. 54–57)

The establishment of this relationship was valuable for Claire's parents, for through it they came to feel that they were not 'in a boat by themselves'. They were able to share in Jill's parents' knowledge of the rare disorder that affected both their children. They were also able to absolve themselves of the guilt that they had felt as a result of feeling that they had 'done the wrong things' in the initial stages of Claire's illness. They now knew that other parents in similar situations had made exactly the same 'mistakes'. Later in the group interview I asked the parents to describe events or people that they had found to be particularly helpful to them. Claire's mother returned to her relationship with Jill's parents:

> **Mother 2:** I have to say that you [Jill's mum] were a great help to us (. . .) and I'm not just saying it because you're there, it's true, just because your daughter has been through it (. . .) that really helped a lot.
> **Mother 4:** It doesn't matter how often the doctors say she will get better, I would have been happier if I'd seen somebody like Jill. (27, p. 58–59)

There was a range of ways in which parents supported each other while in hospital, from 'just listening' to another's problems and anxieties to physically helping with the care of another parent's child. The latter was seen as essentially nurse's work that the parents found themselves doing because nurses were otherwise occupied or unavailable due to staff shortages. Two parents described how they came to take on this role:

> Susan's mum was admitted Thursday or Friday night and she was a wee bit crabbit and that and I said, 'Maybe she needs her bath,' and she says, 'Well, where do I get the stuff?', so I went and got her nappies and towel and cream and everything and she says, 'Which bath do I use?' and I showed her that, I mean, a nurse should have been there. (12, p. 24–25)

> They're short-staffed up in Ward Z: I was up last night with this mother I met in the smoking room and she says, 'Can you come and give me a hand' – there's five bairns down the bottom end and they all scream and keep her wee boy up so she's got to go round the five bairns. . . . There's only two nurses on, a staff nurse and an auxiliary, and I had to help her out the bed with her wee boy, up to the toilet. (. . .) So I went down and patted this wee boy to sleep (. . .) and then this other wee boy started and I'm patting this one and she's patting the other one . . . we were there for about half an hour. (26, Mother 4, p. 13–14)

The most frequently described forms of supportive contact between parents were talking, listening and mutual helping. Parents seemed to sense that this was something of a proscribed activity but one that was widespread nonetheless. As this mother noted:

> It's got a notice up in the Mothers' Unit: 'Please do not discuss your child's illness with other parents as this could lead to distress' and that, but it does go on, I mean, that's **all** that goes on **all the time** is talking about what's wrong with yours and. . . . (25, Mother 1, p. 24)

As with their relationships outwith the hospital, there were varying degrees of closeness among parents. Between some parents the contact was only polite greetings and general enquiries as to how their child was getting on, while for others deeper relationships developed. It was among these closer relationships that most mutual support was evident. Three parents in particular gave accounts of how they had been actively involved in helping other parents through talking with them and perhaps more importantly, by hearing and bearing witness to their stories. One was the mother of Kim, a girl who was comatose as the result of a head injury. Her mother described an incident in the Mothers' Unit that illustrated that parents' concerns were not always exclusively centred upon their own child and that such sharing of experiences and concerns was felt to be beneficial.

> **Mother:** Likes of up in the flat at night when we're all having a cup of tea, right now it's Jean's baby, she's been brought in with a wee hole in her heart (. . .) so they done the operation today and she's blind and she's only 10 months old. So we're trying to comfort Jean; I know there's not much we can say that'll help her but we just sit and let her talk and talk and let her get it out her system.
>
> **PD:** That's interesting, the idea that parents can be, like, a source of support to each other. . . .
>
> **Mother:** Well it was last night that she got the news about her daughter being blind, and all the mothers were up in the unit watching 'The Visit' [a television documentary about a girl's severe head injury and subsequent treatment and rehabilitation], right? and Jean walked in in the middle of it and she was bubbling and crying and talking about Ann being blind and that and then she looked at the television and said, 'Oh God! not more hospitals!' So Lorna turned to Jean and said, 'Aye, but we're trying to watch this to see if we can help Kim's mum with Kim being in a coma,' and of course the lassie was all kinda taken aback, she didn't know. And then she was interested in it and she was asking me about Kim and that took her mind off her baby for a wee while and let her settle down for a wee while. (5, p. 28–29)

Another mother whose daughter had been scalded in a kettle accident described the close relationship and community of caring within which such 'serious talking' could take place. She had become very friendly with a mother [Sandra] from another ward whose child was dying from a condition that had already caused the death of her first child. Another mother [Alice] who knew Sandra very well was coincidentally in the burns unit with her child at this time. The mother explained that

> Alice and I had sort of spoken, you know, just sort of generally, and then she started getting depressed and she didn't want to start crying in front of Sandra, so she started telling me about it and one night she was really upset and said, 'Oh, I really feel like going out,' and I said, 'Well, I'll go with you for a drink,' . . . and so we went and had a couple of drinks, but I started feeling really depressed as well, you know and. . . . Oh God, it was really awful, and actually Sandra came along to see if Alice was all right 'cos she was worried about her and so we were all talking, but it was really . . . she wasn't . . . Sandra wasn't as depressed as Alice about it and at one point I

was getting really depressed, you know, 'cos she was such a lovely girl, and what a shame it was to lose two the same way (. . .) and that sort of contact was really close, and really quite emotional. (10, p. 26–27)

These parents' relationships had developed from generally polite but superficial contact to ones where more meaningful but painful feelings could be shared. It is perhaps significant that this talking and listening had to take place outside the hospital as Alice had 'really felt like going out'. This may have been due to her feeling that she needed to 'get away from it all' for a short while. An alternative interpretation is that these relationships developed more easily, with talking and listening occurring more naturally in normal social settings rather than in a paediatric ward or Mothers' Unit sitting room.

In addition to listening to and talking with other parents, some parents would encourage and boost the morale of others. One mother described how other parents in the Mothers' Unit had done this for her:

There's a few mammies says to me up in the unit, 'By God, you're doing a great job, Christine, I don't know where you get your strength from, day after day, week after week . . . where do you get your strength from, how can you keep going?' So I says, 'Well, if you give up, she'll give up. You've got to keep going for her sake.' (5, p. 52–53)

Similarly, a father described an incident where he had tried to reassure two parents who were sitting, clearly distressed, in the ward corridor outside the burns unit's intensive care unit:

We'd been in for three weeks and Gordon's mum was sitting out there (. . .) and I says, 'What's wrong?' . . . She said, 'My wee boy's in the bath, he's all burnt and that and I can't go in and face him.' (. . .) So I looked in and I seen wee Gordon sitting there, just . . . and I thought, what's she all worried about? . . . but I suppose when it's your own it's different, and I went back through and says, 'He looks great!' I says, 'He's not bad.' I couldn't see his feet, how bad they were, but he wasn't crying . . . I came back out and I explained all about Alex [his son who had been very severely scalded all over his body] and what had happened to my wee boy and how bad he was. I wasn't bumming [boasting] about it but just trying to explain how good the doctors was, and says, 'Why don't you go through?' (. . .) So I popped my head into the unit and Staff Nurse Patricia was in and I said, 'Is it all right if I take the laddie's mum and dad through?' (. . .) so I took them through and said, 'That's him in there and he's doing fine,' and . . . (. . .) I could have said a lot more about infection and that but it wasn't my place . . . but just to give the bare necessities from start to finish (. . .) from somebody that's actually been there . . . nobody told us, we had to find out for ourselves. (18, p. 60–61)

To professionals this may seem a crude and insensitive approach, for this father had effectively said to these parents that their worries were relatively minor when compared with the severity of his son's injuries and that their anxieties were therefore out of proportion. He did however make the significant point that any talk of appropriate levels of distress was itself inappropriate because 'when it's your own, it's different'. This father used his experiences to support and reassure these other parents who were coming into this strange and terrifying situation in the same way that he himself had done three weeks earlier. Interestingly, in a focus group, Gordon's parents mentioned that this meeting with Alex's father in the corridor had been of real help to them:

> **Gordon's mother**: You need somebody else with you, 'cos if it wasn't for you and your man that night when Gordon came in I don't know where we'd be today 'cos we were in some mess. . . .
> **Gordon's father:** Oh, aye, you need somebody else.
> **Gordon's mother:** . . . well, just going through what happened to theirs.
> **Alex's mother:** . . . like, she [Gordon's mother] was up to high doh and Alex was in the intensive care at the time and Jack [her husband] had seen her bairn and said, 'Look, my bairn's lying in there and if you could see him you would have something to worry about. Your bairn's all right, where [if] they [the nurses] just went and left him there himself.
> **Gordon's mother:** It pulled us up a bit. (25, p. 22–23, 25)

One feature of this account was the absence of any mention of nursing staff attention paid to Gordon's parents as they sat outside the treatment room 'in some mess' and 'up to high doh'. This raises the question of whether **any** caring attentions, perhaps from a nurse, would have been appreciated or whether there was something very specific about Alex's father's intervention that was particularly valued. It seemed from the accounts that Gordon's mother particularly appreciated the reassurance that came from someone who had personal experience of what they were then going through. Another important element seemed to have been Alex's father's emphasis on hope and positive messages. He had told them that their child's scalds were comparatively minor, that the doctors were particularly good, that he was doing fine and that this experience was a journey, a traumatic one perhaps, but nonetheless one that had an end.

Parents' accounts suggested that the relationships that existed among parents were of greater importance than nurses had previously assumed. Far from being involved in insensitive gossip, cliquishness or conspiracy, parents through their quiet presencing were bearing witness to each other's distress and providing more valuable mutual support than they were perhaps able to articulate.

5.6.2 Difficulties experienced in relationships between parents

It would be wrong to romanticize the relationships that existed between parents as being entirely supportive and mutually satisfactory. Parents emphasized that, in hospital as in the outside world, there were people whom they liked and befriended and others whom they disliked and avoided. The common bond of being parents of a hospitalized child did not overcome this aspect of normal social functioning. As one mother explained:

> I suppose it's just the same as anywhere else, there are people that you will be able to talk to and get on with and there will be people that you will not. It's not that you are all in the same boat really because you can be in the same boat with someone and still not have anything in common with them and not be able to talk to them. (17, p. 66–67)

Parents described other parents who were unsupportive and even positively annoying. Parents who were described as being 'nosy' or insensitive at an especially traumatic time were particularly criticized. This was possibly the rationale behind the caution printed in the Mothers' Unit information booklet, that 'gossip about your own or other's children can distress some people'.

Such distress was often described as being the result of parents disregarding or failing to observe the very carefully balanced interactional synchrony that existed in the communication and relationships between parents. A delicate social balance operated between the expression of concern for another parent's wellbeing and that of their child and what parents deemed to be nosiness and insensitivity. Parents' initial encounters were usually restricted to very general and diplomatic questions that were phrased as simple expressions of concern. One mother described this:

> I've got to know a few of the mothers here, but because we've just said hello for a few days and then they'll say, 'How's the wee one?' . . . but not ask delving questions. (17, p. 65)

Another mother explained in more detail how this balance was achieved:

> You don't ask what's wrong with their child, but sort of say, how are they, . . . 'cos if they're not very great [well], that can be quite awkward . . . and you just develop from that and if somebody comes and sits next to you and . . . you just say, 'How's things?', a really general thing . . . they can either take it to mean themselves or . . . and if they don't mention the child then you never sort of ask 'cos it could mean that there's something . . . (10, p. 28)

This account revealed the sensitivity required if parents were to achieve this balance between the expression of concerned interest and insensitive prying. When parents described the occasions when they felt that others had got this wrong and had been insensitive, it was clear that this was the cause of some distress. The mother quoted above continued in her account, to describe such an occasion when her friend Sandra, whose child was dying, had gone down to the parents' coffee and smoking room:

> This couple, they said, 'How is she?' and she said, 'Not so great,' and shaking her head a bit. 'Oh, what's the matter?' . . . and she said, you know, 'Oh I don't really want to talk about it,' shook her head, waved her hand and

that . . . but they just persisted, you know, and she just walked out 'cos if she hadn't she would have just totally. . . (. . .) There can be a lot of friction if people are insensitive and some people do, they just say ,'Oh, what's your child in with? How did it happen?' Some people are just too nosy (. . .) even if the child's not going to die, (. . .) you get some visitors, even, and you hear them saying, 'What's the matter with that one over there?' (. . .) just insensitive and nosy and it drives me up the wall. (10, p. 29–30)

The mother of a seriously ill baby described a similar situation. In this extract she clearly brought out some of the difficulties involved in being the parent of a sick child in a public arena, where once private concerns could be pressed into becoming common property.

Once I felt terrible because another little boy was brought into the unit from another hospital and his auntie, I think, was sitting down beside me in the corridor and she was a perfectly nice woman but Jamie was having a trauma at the time and she said, 'Is that your wee baby that's in there?' . . . 'Wee boy or wee girl?' I said, 'It's a wee boy' . . . trying to give one word answers, just to say . . . you know I didn't want to say, 'Leave me alone!' . . . She said, 'How old is he?' . . . 'Three months.' . . . 'Is he all right?' . . . and I really wanted to turn round and say, 'Well he's not in intensive care 'cos he's got a cold!' . . . but I actually managed to . . . . . . and I just said, 'I really don't want to talk about it, I'm sorry', and afterwards I felt pretty rotten (. . .) because then you feel guilty unless you're the type of person that enjoys being rude (. . .) but at times like that you're not yourself, you can't be expected to be. (17, p. 62–63)

This mother described a similar finely balanced interactional comportment when she described how she had found it very difficult to speak to another mother.

There's a little baby in the unit just now with Jamie who's . . . looks just like Jamie did when he was first in there, if not worse, 'cos he . . . his brain seems to be affected. . . . I don't know what's wrong 'cos I haven't asked 'cos I know how I felt when people asked about Jamie, but I just don't feel that I could speak to his mother . . . you know, because I know how I felt and nobody could say anything. . . . . . . 'cos I saw her today, it was the funniest thing. . . . I watched her sitting beside her little boy and I thought, that was me three weeks ago, and I found that I can't find it in myself to say anything to her, because I felt that I should . . . from deep down be able to find something to say to her because I had been there, I had done that (. . .) but I couldn't. It's not that I had forgotten what it's like. It's probably 'cos I remembered all too well what it's like and I saw her and I thought, you're just . . . if I could just have sent it, sort of . . . transferred it by telepathy, I would have, but I knew there was nothing to say. . . . I just wanted to say, 'I've been there, I've done this . . . it's just absolute hell.' (17, p. 71–73)

Seeing this other mother created dilemmas for Jamie's mother. She recognized that the other mother was suffering as she herself had done. She wanted to help by sharing her experiences and letting her know that here was someone who had 'been there' and really did know what she was going through. She was constrained, however, by her memories of how she herself had felt when anyone had tried to comfort her in similar ways. Timing seemed very important in such a situation, in that Jamie's mum wanted very much to help this other mother but realized that this was not the right time, regardless of how sensitively she might have done it.

5.7 CONCLUDING COMMENTS

I have illuminated parents' lived experiences through a discussion of the network of relationships within which such experiences were embedded. The nurse–parent relationship could be both static and dynamic. In this respect, the passage of time and the length of a parent's stay in the ward were found to be important factors. However, I suggest that significant and positive developments in the nurse–parent relationship were not attributable solely to the passage of time.

Other important factors were at work that helped to shape the nature of this relationship. For example it seemed important that the nurse was afforded opportunities to transcend first impressions and get to know the person of the parent. It seemed similarly important that the parent was allowed to learn something of the person behind the professional nurse. The importance of nurses' caring practices and approaches allowed the relationship between parent and nurse to progress from an impersonally professional basis to a more emotionally and personally involved connected relationship.

Nurses have found the ideas of the philosopher Martin Buber particularly useful in understanding human relationships (Roach, 1987; Bishop and Scudder, 1990). Buber, in his 'I–Thou' dialogues (Buber, 1958), differentiated between what he called I–Thou and I–It relationships. I–It relationships are relationships that we have with things and are characterized by utilitarian concerns, detachment, manipulation and the sense that while 'it' may influence me, I do not influence 'it'. The parents' and nurses' accounts suggested that this was the predominant mode of relationship between them. Parents' stories spoke of being outside, of being the object of nurses' attentions, of not feeling truly involved and understood. Nurses spoke of parents' characteristics, and their usefulness. Recall also that nurses' accounts described how parents' personalities affected them, but not how they mutually affected parents. In contrast to I–It relationships, I–Thou relationships are unique, intimate, personal and mutual. There is a fusion of concerns in I–Thou relationships that transform the I and Thou to a We.

While Buber's distinctions between human relationships are useful in helping to understand the nature of the nurse–parent relationship there are two other dimensions that need to be acknowledged. The first is that the nurses were involved, not in a dyadic but in a triadic relationship. Relations with the parents cannot be separated from relations with the child. Secondly, nurses were expected to be involved not in one close, personal relationship but in several. Bishop and Scudder (1990) have recognized the need to interpret Buber's ideas within the specific context of a practice discipline such as nursing. They suggest that, even when nurses are carrying out routine procedures and interactions, they can still bring an I–Thou dimension to the relationship by recognizing and preserving the patient's unique personhood. Bishop and Scudder (1990) also make the useful point that a personal relationship is not incompatible with an organizational structure or routine. Neither is it a purely private or individual arrangement. They suggest that 'a personal relationship is one in which I respond to a particular person as he is present to me in ways which express my way of being with that person' (Bishop and Scudder 1990, p. 149). I suggest that this explanation would have a resonance for both the parents who described how they had felt cared for and cared about by particular nurses, and those nurses themselves.

It is significant in relation to this chapter's discussion of parents' relationships that one of the few papers that mentioned this aspect of living-in was written by a medical sociologist who had actually lived-in with her own child who had been scalded. Webb (1977) argued that mothers formed a collective 'safety valve' where issues could be discussed in an open way that was not possible with staff. This occurred, for example, when parents swapped 'horror stories' of staff mistakes, changes in treatment plans and other difficulties that the parents faced.

This was also true of the mothers in this present study who often found the company of and contact with other mothers to be extremely valuable. The parents were similarly involved in endless discussions about their children and their treatments and progress. This was so obvious and widespread that it seemed that mothers were completely ignoring the hospital's advice that such 'gossip' should be avoided, but this was not so. I suggest that the mothers largely ignored this advice because **it** ignored the subtle and complex ways in which parents related and communicated their shared concerns, joys and anxieties. The illness or injury of their child was so overwhelmingly present in this situation and such an inalienable part of their being as parents that it was inconceivable to parents that they could pass a day without the subject being raised. This advice also ignored the ways in which such discussions among parents were beneficial in allowing them to care for each other. As they shared experiences and concerns, this allowed them to 'set up the possibility of giving help and receiving help' (Benner and Wrubel, 1989, p. 4).

The parents were well aware of the fact that 'gossip' could be distressing but did not see this as being the result of talking about their child's treatment. Rather they saw this as part of a more general lack of sensitivity and inappropriate timing on the part of others. Some parents seemed not to realize that this was not the time to ask that question or did not appreciate that at that moment another parent simply wanted to be left alone.

Webb (1977) also argued that parents as a group had no coherent identity and would never, for example, 'use their group identity as a basis for collective action'. She also claimed that 'in relations with the staff, the individualistic nature of your interests was stressed. Each cubicle was a different "scene" in the total ward drama; to intervene on behalf of some other actor was as inappropriate as making an entrance on to the wrong stage-play' (Webb, 1977, p. 185). Webb was clearly surprised and disappointed that this was so but I argue that it would be more surprising were this not the case.

The parents' accounts suggested that there may have been some shared group identity based upon their sense of 'all being in the same boat'. They were, after all, live-in parents of children in hospital. This however was an insufficiently strong or discrete force to provide any basis for what Webb calls 'collective action'. While Webb argued that it was the staff who stressed 'the individualistic nature' of parents' interests, this ignores the wishes of the parents themselves. Staff certainly emphasized the individuality of children and their families, for not to do so would quickly have led to charges that they were providing institutional care which batch-processed people with no regard for their particular circumstances.

However it was also parents themselves who demanded that they and their child were treated as individuals. They were sensitive to and critical of staff who treated them as just another scald, or cleft lip, or appendectomy and who failed to provide care that recognized and catered for their child's particular idiosyncrasies, likes and dislikes. It would be wrong, however, to polarize this question as being a stark choice between a collective or individual identity since parents' accounts suggest that both were desired. An important finding in this respect, which will be developed further in Chapter 6, is that through nurses' caring practices this could be achieved.

Parents expressed a strong desire to feel that they were not alone with their child's illness that there were others who had experienced this trauma, and who had 'gone through what they were going through'. Here, a collective identity based upon the child's unique illness or injury seemed especially important to parents. This gave a clearer focus to their sharing than did the more general bond that existed between all parents of a sick child in hospital. While the latter was invoked to suggest more general changes that would be of universal benefit, such as improved living facilities, the disease-specific sharing seemed to provide something of a more uniquely personal value.

Concluding discussion | 6

6.1 INTRODUCTION

This research had three main purposes. I sought to understand the lived experiences of parents who stayed in hospital with their child, to gain a deeper understanding of the experiences and perceptions of paediatric nurses as these related to their relationships with parents and to explore the nature of the relationships that developed between parents and between parents and nurses. Here I review what was attempted, what was learned and suggest further questions raised by the study.

First, I briefly reflect on the philosophical approach that underpinned the study. I then review and extend the discussion of the major themes that have emerged from the interpretive analysis of the participants' accounts. Next I outline, in relation to the original aims, what the study has contributed to knowledge regarding the lived experiences of live-in parents and their relationships with paediatric nurses. Finally I discuss the implications of the study for paediatrics and for nursing.

6.2 THE RESEARCH PHILOSOPHY AND APPROACH REVIEWED

Traditional, formal education has been criticized both by researchers (Allen, 1985; Bordo, 1986; McMahon, 1991) and particularly effectively through the allegorical fiction of Pirsig (1974), for sustaining a view of scholarship and analysis as being synonymous with the production of closure, proven truths, detached abstract theory, unequivocal meanings and unassailable knowledge. This view of scholarship and, in particular, the relationship between data, description and theory is untenable within this study's philosophical approach (Heidegger, 1962; Taylor, 1985a; b; Benner, 1990b; Van Manen, 1990)

Interpretive phenomenology was used to offer a range of understandings that are essentially hermeneutic. There is an emphasis on what Husserl (1982) called 'the things themselves'; the essences of the lived experiences described by parents and nurses. In order to achieve this I have described the contextual meaning of a wide range of parents' and nurses' everyday actions, thoughts and under-standings. While trying to remain true to participants' everyday understandings, I have also brought further horizons of meaning to bear on the participants' accounts.

6.3 MAJOR THEMES OF THE STUDY

One of the most difficult interpretive decisions to make in qualitative research is determining which stories to tell and which to reasonably set aside from a body of data which is too vast and rich to be able to include everything. The pheno-menological researcher's involvement allows the openness to dialogue, puzzles, possibilities and questions necessary for such interpretive decisions to be made. Here I review what I consider to be the study's major themes and implications.

6.3.1 The nature of being a live-in parent in hospital

This research suggests that previous attempts to understand live-in parents in primarily functional terms of roles and responsibilities (Meadow, 1969; Knafl et al., 1988) have given us a very limited insight into the meaning of their lived experiences. Drawing on the work of Heidegger (1962) and Benner and Wrubel (1989) I have followed an ontological turn that better uncovers the nature of being human and, in this specific instance, of being a live-in parent.

(a) The ontological sense of being a live-in parent

In trying to understand the lived experience of being the resident parent of a hospitalized child, I believe that it is necessary to step back a little and consider first what is the more fundamental question: what does it mean to be a parent? This step is important because live-in parents have a background of cultural and caring practices and understandings that they bring to their new situation.

Being a parent can be viewed from several different perspectives. Biological, ethnological and psychoanalytic theories stress the inherent and instinctual drives that cast motherhood as both natural and almost a biological inevitability (Boulton, 1983). Social theories view parenthood as a socially constructed job, social role and set of skills to be performed on or with children (La Rossa, 1986). Both biologically and socially based theories of parenthood tend to focus upon parenting behaviours rather than the lived experiences of parents themselves. Even when the need is expressly acknowledged that parents' experiences are important, this is often taken to mean 'women's subjective experiences' (Boulton, 1983). It is typical here for subjective to be taken as synonymous with either a private world or that which is not objective.

The phenomenological approach used here, influenced by the work of Heidegger (1962) and Benner (1985a; 1989; 1990b), attempts to dissolve this distinction between subjective and objective worlds. This approach is based upon an assumption that meanings are not private, designative and possessed, but rather common, relational and constitutive of the person (Taylor, 1985a). Although recent phenomenological and interpretive studies have examined the lived experiences of parents, the question of what it means to be a parent remains elusive (Bergum, 1988; Ruddick, 1989; Van Manen, 1990).

The parents' accounts here suggested however, that even the sum of the 'roles' and 'skills' of parenting could not adequately capture the meaning of being a parent and especially of being a live-in parent in hospital. This became particularly evident as parents tried to explain how they felt about the experience. Although they could discuss and describe particular aspects of their being live-in parents, for many the more primordial question of 'What is it like to be the resident parent of a sick child?' was literally beyond description.

I propose that nurses need to see being a parent as an ontological relationship, as a particular way of being-in-the-world with a child. Viewing parenthood as fundamentally a question of being helps us to see how parents are parents in a 'world-defining' sense (Rubin, 1984; Benner and Wrubel, 1989, p. 82). Again, this is a notion of meaning where the child constitutes the parent's world rather than where parents are merely designated as being the people who have a child. The parents' child was not simply the **object** of their parental work, attention, care and concern. Their child was an inalienable part of themselves and their world, and *vice versa*.

This approach to understanding the nature of being a parent helps to make more comprehensible the experiences of the parents who said that they wished that the accident could have happened to them, or that they could have undergone the operation in place of their child or who asked that their skin rather than their child's be used for grafts.

This ontological view of being a parent allows an interpretive understanding of the themes that arose from the parents' accounts. For example, when I asked parents why they chose to live-in with their child, many parents seemed genuinely not to understand that this was any kind of rational choice or decision. They could not conceive of a situation or world, albeit a temporary one, where they would not be staying with their child at this particular time.

Parents also described how they were unable to articulate how they felt about a particularly traumatic aspect of their child's hospitalization. When this occurred they often explained that unless you were a parent who had gone through a similar experience, you would never be able to understand 'what it was like'. These parents would have understood Van Manen's (1990, p. 61) observation that parenting 'is something primordial which defies literal language and precise definition'.

Further support for this ontological understanding of parenthood was given in Chapter 5. Recall that parents described how they believed that they received more understanding care from nurses who were themselves parents and whose 'whole manner' was consequently qualitatively different. This understanding of the meaning of being a parent was echoed by some nurses who had returned to nursing after having children. They claimed that becoming parents had markedly changed their understanding of how live-in parents 'must feel'. They also described how their paediatric nursing practice had changed as a result of the greater empathy and insight which they now had through becoming parents. These nurses had discovered that understanding is a way of being rather than of merely cognitively knowing (Heidegger, 1962; Gadamer, 1975).

(b) The situated meaning of being a live-in parent

Live-in parents were parents in an unfamiliar public arena at a time of great personal and family stress. For these reasons it is necessary to consider the situation of the live-in parent. Although previous mention was made in Chapter 2 of the use of 'situation' in its Heideggerian sense, it is useful to briefly review this.

Parents were indeed in a strange and unfamiliar environment within the ward, but the term 'environment' has been properly criticized for its restricted focus upon the physical features of a place (Chopoorian, 1986; Benner and Wrubel, 1989). Drawing upon Heidegger (1962), Benner and Wrubel (1989, p. 80) note that 'situation implies a social definition and meaningfulness'. This is an important distinction as it stresses the importance of people and their concerns and interpretations. Heidegger wrote of places and spaces as functions of concern, that is, they are places **for** something (MacQuarrie, 1972). Other phenomenologists (Bollnow, 1961; Seamon, 1984; Van Manen, 1990) have given insightful descriptions of the existential quality of 'lived space' or 'spatiality' in relation to various spaces in our lives.

How then were the live-in parents 'in' the situation? This question makes more sense when we consider Heidegger's observation that human existence or being-in-the-world 'is not to be thought of as a characteristic of objects spatially located with respect to other objects' (Dreyfus, 1991, p. 40). In other words, a parent was not 'in' the ward in the same way that a bed or locker was 'in' the ward. The crucial difference here, as Dreyfus (1991) notes, is that the former implies an existential involvement whereas the latter suggests only inclusion.

This study's findings suggest that parents were often 'in' their situation in ways that were characterized by a lack of involvement, confusion, uncertainty and anxiety. Benner and Wrubel (1989) have observed that a person's interpretation of their situation is neither a wholly private nor simple free choice. Interpretations are more shared and communal. In this study, I have presented an understanding of social phenomena as being co-created by parents and nurses. Such an understanding, in the Gadamerian sense previously described, involves working towards a fusion of horizons, where the participant's horizon of understanding fuses with that of the researcher or interpreter. The following discussion attempts to develop such an understanding of the parents' situation.

Parents were used to being parents with their child at home and it is useful first to consider the situated meaning of 'home'. Home is a private domain where parents carry out most of their child-care practices and a great deal of other 'women's work' (Oakley, 1974a; b). In proposing this concept of parenting as a mostly private, home-centred activity, I acknowledge Ruddick's point that 'mothers do not work in private. They are always in public' (Ruddick, 1989, p. 35).

However, while it is true that parenting is an increasingly visible practice, as is clear, for example, from the proliferation of popular magazines devoted to instructing people 'how to become a better parent', I maintain that its most sensitive practices, such as showing overt love and disciplining, are still essentially practices restricted to the home.

Home is also where parents live with immediate family and where they can 'be themselves'. In order to 'feel at home' where they can be themselves, the concepts of control and privacy are central, as community nurses have long recognized (McIntosh, 1979). Usually, parents choose who, if anyone, is allowed to enter their home and, once there, visitors usually respect certain territorial boundaries. For example, a visiting friend would be unlikely to enter your bedroom uninvited. As Allan and Crow (1989, p. 4) note, 'being in a private place is a central part of what it means to be "at home"'. Being at home also carries a sense of security, familiarity and freedom from anxiety or worry. Being at home in a place means being able to relax. The home is also the place where we return to after any periods spent in public. Home also carries wider connotations of warmth and comfort (Heller, 1984) and a sense of values and good that we may return to after having left, the sense of 'coming home' or 'back to our roots'. Van Manen (1990, p. 102) reminds us that home is much more than just a physical environment when he observes that our feelings for homeless people are so strong because 'we sense that there is a deeper tragedy involved than merely not having a roof over one's head'.

How then did the situated meaning of the ward or Mother's Unit differ from the live-in parents' familiar home? I suggest that the parents were 'parenting in public', in that they were expected to be parents but under the scrutiny of professionals and other parents. Parents were now in a situation where even previously private child-care practices were to be in public view. The difficulties that this caused for parents were highlighted in their discussions of discipline in Chapter 2.

While parents at home lived with family and could develop social relations with others on a voluntary basis, they were now living with strangers, both nurses and other live-in parents. Parents who were sleeping in the hospital's Mothers' Unit seemed to find this most difficult. How the parent was engaged in the situation inextricably influenced their interpretations and self-understandings. For example, if their child's illness was particularly severe or even life-threatening, parents were so concerned with their child that they were grateful for anywhere to sleep and privacy would be of lesser importance. For other parents, sleeping in a small two-bedded room with another mother created a sense of violated privacy and enforced contact. A further concern regarding lack of privacy was that parents had no 'private place', in either the geographical or emotional sense, where they could go if they were particularly upset, crying or wanted to 'just be alone'.

Parents also described how the ward had a different sense of time and rhythm from home. This can be more readily understood when we consider that the structure and content of the live-in parent's day were now so different, as Chapter 4 showed. For example, live-in parents described the slow passage of time and the sense of merely reacting to the timetables of others, whereas at home such timetables would have been under their control. Parents' natural anxieties and fears for their child meant that the ward was not a situation where they could feel at home in the sense of being relaxed and carefree. Significantly here, when parents described how they tried to relax they spoke of 'getting away from the ward for a bit', by going along to a nearby bar or perhaps going home for a day.

Since parents were neither at home physically nor existentially, the question arises as to whose place the ward was. Nurses did not live there but worked there, while parents did not 'work' there but (temporarily) lived there. It seems clear from the previous chapters that, while the ward may not have been the nurses' actual home, it shared many of the characteristics of home for them, if not for parents. Nurses were clearly more 'at home' in the ward than were parents. The ward was home to a set of professional values and practices and, as Chapters 3 and 4 showed, parents approached these with the circumspection of a guest or visitor. Parents also treated the ward's areas as a visitor would, by seeking permission initially to enter the 'host's' areas such as linen cupboards, bathing rooms, toy cupboards and, of course, the ward kitchen.

Chapter 4 showed that nurses used a home analogy as a well-meaning attempt to make parents feel more relaxed and at home while living-in. However, as the previous discussion has shown, it was difficult for live-in parents to experience the ward in such a way as to make them feel at home. As I would stress, it was often the seemingly trivial encounters that were most revealing of the participants' lived experiences. If this study shows anything, it is that there are no such things as 'little things'. In this respect, it was hard to see how parents could feel at home if they were not allowed to go and make a slice of toast in the kitchen, walk into the ward in a nightdress or watch their favourite soap-opera on television.

To return to the phenomenological sense of 'lived space' or 'situation', I suggest that, just as motorways, for example, are not places 'to be' but rather means to enable us to get to somewhere (Van Manen, 1990), perhaps the paediatric ward was not a place where parents could comfortably **be** with their child. There was support for this interpretation in the accounts of the parents who spoke of their stay as being somehow 'unreal', an 'unnatural existence', and where they were 'just there'. The nurses too may have sensed this when they discussed parents who had been 'in too long' and who 'needed to get out'.

One of the clear findings of this study is that parents, and this must be recognized as meaning almost exclusively mothers, were conscious of a need to be perceived as a 'good mother' in the eyes of their child, their family, professional staff, other parents and indeed themselves. For live-in parents, this became a moral and social endeavour as well as a practical one. Ruddick (1989, p. 31), in her study of maternal thinking, has noted that 'an idealized figure of the Good Mother casts a long shadow on many actual mothers' lives', and the mothers in this study were no exception.

Parents were expected to 'perform' the most complex and delicate of social balancing acts. They had to be demonstrably caring and concerned for their child yet had to avoid giving the impression of being over-protective, over-anxious or 'neurotic'. Parents had to show an interest in all aspects of their child's care, treatment and progress yet had to avoid being a nuisance or asker of repeated or 'stupid' questions. Parents had to show a willingness to participate in their child's care yet had to avoid 'taking over' from the nurses. Parents had to be there at the child's bedside yet had to avoid being in the way. Parents had to show that they were competent care providers for their child while acknowledging that the professionals knew best. Parents were also encouraged to do whatever they would do for their child at home yet were expected to adhere to the occasionally arbitrary and conflicting rules of the ward or hospital.

These 'performance criteria' were largely achieved by parents, despite their being in the poorest of circumstances to 'perform'. Despite these tensions, parents did manage to endure living-in with their child for the duration of their hospitalization. During the period of fieldwork I was unaware of any live-in parent who had 'given up' and returned home. However, such a yardstick of success is clearly inadequate and would reveal nothing of parents' important experiences, participation and involvement with their child's care during their stay.

(c) Being in the situation: involvement and control

Live-in parents had to adapt to a situation where they were negotiating and adapting to being participants in the care of their own child. This contrasts with a possible alternative view, that it was nurses who were in fact participating in the care of the parents' child. This difference was more than merely linguistic and raises important issues of 'ownership' of and responsibility for the child.

The parents described the difficulties that they faced as they entered both the domain and the discourse of perceived child-care experts. They also highlighted their diminished sense of control over and involvement in the aspects of their child's care where they had previously felt most comfortable, for example in their accounts of discipline and basic mothering.

The parents' and nurses' accounts have shown that they acknowledged legitimate differences in relation to 'areas of ownership' of the child. Nurses frequently pointed out that there were many aspects of the child's care that should be the preserve primarily of parents. Similarly, parents entering the hospital were well aware that they were not doctors or nurses and indeed in their accounts they stressed that their sick child was 'in the best place' where the staff would know what to do for them. The parents showed no desire to take control of their child's surgical operation or the prescribing of their medication. This supports Benner and Wrubel's view that 'when a committed couple must weather an extreme illness of a partner or parents must face a devastating illness of their child, autonomy, mastery, control, and rationality are not the salient issues' (Benner and Wrubel, 1989, p. 84).

Put bluntly, at this particular time the parents had more important concerns in mind. However, as the immediate crisis or extreme situation passed, concerns such as control, understanding and involvement became more important for parents. I argue that it is inadequate to view issues of involvement and control primarily in terms of a polarization between parents and hospital professionals and between technical care and parental care. Parents and nurses often experienced conflict in relation to 'who knows best for the child' or 'who should be doing what for the child'. However, the following discussion will show that parents' and nurses' experiences of involvement and participation were more complex than traditional conceptions of power and control have acknowledged.

Chapter 4 showed that parent participation was a subtle, dynamic yet frequently unarticulated social phenomena created by the expectations, approaches and strategies of both nurses and parents. Previous studies in this field have tended to characterize parent participation in stark, confrontational terms of power, control and professional dominance, for example Webb (1977), Robinson (1985) and Beuf (1979). Such studies commonly envisioned power as an external force, possessed by and emanating from a central source, in this case, the institution of the hospital and its agents of social control, the nurses. I suggest that these participants' accounts support an alternative interpretation of power that affords a deeper understanding of the nature of parents' experiences, and in particular of their participation and involvement.

The conceptualization of power as an external possession of others has been most successfully challenged by Foucault (1980) who argued that modern power is more subtle yet more effective than earlier power. Unlike previously centralized systems of power, modern power is characteristically 'capillary' in that it exists not in 'agents of social control', but everywhere throughout the social body, down to the smallest 'micropractices'. Thus power is not so much something which a consultant, ward sister or staff nurse 'has' and which a parent 'has not'. Rather, power is present in all aspects of everyday social life, in all of our practices, habits and gestures.

The implications of a Foucauldian view of power relationships are that we can most usefully focus not upon power itself, or upon 'the balance of power between nurses and parents' as Callery and Smith (1991) suggested, but on how power is exercised (Nettleton, 1991). Foucault showed that with the development of modern power there was less reliance upon grand official or state gestures and displays of power. Instead, there developed an increasing surveillance of the population in general and especially within institutions such as prisons, schools and hospitals (Foucault, 1977; 1980).

An illustration of this idea relevant to nursing would be the disappearance of the 'Matron's round'. Here, Matron, as the embodiment of power over nurses, would tour the whole hospital to check on individual patients and the performance of nurses. Now, such surveillance has been devolved to a range of managers and to a large extent to the ward nurses who are encouraged to monitor themselves, in the name of professional responsibility and autonomy.

Foucault developed his idea of 'the gaze' from two surveillance practices (Fraser, 1989). The first was the synoptic visibility of the Panopticon, named after Bentham's cartwheel-like design for a prison-type structure that allowed for constant observation of the inmate from a central 'hub'. Also influential was individualizing visibility, characterized by professional and official observation of individuals and the compilation of increasing amounts of detail concerning all aspects of the lives of those who were now 'cases'.

What is the relevance of Foucault's concept of 'the gaze' for this study and for paediatric nursing? I am less concerned here with the synoptic visibility of parents within the ward. It is true that the traditional Nightingale ward, of which the wards in the study hospital were a modernized version, was a variation of the Panopticon that was designed to allow uninterrupted visibility. I cannot however develop this as a more concrete analogy. Disregarding the architectural differences between the ward and the cell of the Panopticon, there was another crucial difference. The inmates of the Panopticon were never to know when they were being observed, but must always **feel** that they might be. The parents, however, did know that they were being observed because of the visible presence of nurses and other parents. However, it is important to remember that, as Chapter 3 showed, parents did sense that they were being 'watched' and judged. Another important difference between the ward and the Panopticon is that the nurses themselves described their awareness of being the objects of the parents' gaze. They too were under surveillance and scrutiny.

Foucault's idea of the individualizing gaze seems more useful for an understanding of how power relations between nurses and parents operated. Chapter 3 showed how parents fell under a 'normalizing gaze' (Foucault, 1977) within the ward through which they were observed, classified and judged as good parents or otherwise. Such surveillance or 'observation of the patient' has a long history in nursing.

Foucault (1977, p. 184) argues that this normalizing gaze is 'a surveillance that makes it possible to qualify, to classify and to punish'. To illustrate Foucault's point that power is best understood through practices, however small, rather than inferred from attitudes or beliefs, recall, for example, the importance of the ward kitchen for parents and nurses. Parents could, as was shown, be granted access to this usually excluded area by being classified as 'sensible enough' or by being, in Foucault's (1977) words, 'docile, useful bodies'. Parents also received the punishment of nurses' censure for illegitimate trespass into the kitchen. Not surprisingly, perhaps, Craik (1989, p. 48) chose to describe the domestic kitchen as 'the panopticon of the modern home'.

There was a further dimension of Foucault's analysis of power maintained by the seemingly innocuous use of observation and scrutiny that had a resonance with the parents' accounts. Taking another practice, this time the parents' disciplinary approaches, it was shown in Chapter 2 that parents were acutely self-aware as to whether their disciplinary style was acceptable within the professional (ward) context of idealized expert care. The parents also tried to adapt and reform their disciplinary practices to conform to the professional disciplinary ethos of the ward. My point is supported by Foucault's observation that where the disciplinary and normative gaze is perceived to be pervasive, that the objects of this gaze will effectively survey themselves. As Foucault explained: 'He who is subject to a field of visibility, and who knows it, assumes responsibility for the constraints of power, he makes them play spontaneously upon himself; he inscribes in himself the power relation in which he simultaneously plays both roles he becomes the principle of his own subjection' (Foucault, 1977, p. 203).

Foucault's conception of the gaze is valuable in developing an understanding of parents' experiences and power relationships but this conception of an omnipresent capillary power poses problems for those who seek change and improvement. Silverman (1985; 1987; 1989) has frequently argued that the human sciences and reformist, liberal and enlightenment movements are unable to challenge power because they are so deeply implicated in its maintenance. So, has a Foucauldian turn led to a brick wall where nurses can only respond to the negative and alienating aspects of power and surveillance by accepting the status quo? I believe that the accounts of the parents and nurses in this study show that this situation is not so pessimistic as Foucault has claimed.

At this point it is useful to consider this discussion more clearly in the light of the understandings and possibilities raised by this study. I suggest that there is a valuable connection to be made between Foucault's 'multiple points of resistance' (Gubrium and Silverman, 1989), his emphasis on practices over belief systems (Fraser, 1989), and the work of nursing scholars such as Benner (1984; 1988) who have focused upon the primacy of nurses' caring practices. Specifically, this turn in thinking allows for an examination of nurses' specific caring practices, and to consider how these practices may have constituted transformative interventions at particular 'points of resistance'. In other words, I suggest that power relations between nurses and parents can be transformed for the better, and indeed often were for the parents in this study.

Support for this proposition was particularly evident in Chapter 3 where it was shown that the nature of relations was changed by nurses being able to 'get to know the person of the parent'. Similarly in Chapter 5 it was shown that parents valued relationships that developed from the more hierarchical professional–parent basis to a personal relationship characterized more by mutuality and friendship. This is not a simplistic suggestion that nurses 'gave up' power to parents but an understanding that nurses can use their power to empower parents in specific ways that are best viewed as part of a wider discussion of caring within the nurse–parent relationship.

First, however, a criticism must be raised of Foucault's analysis of power relations that has a direct relevance to this discussion. As Fraser (1989) has noted, Foucault's suggestion that power relations can be challenged at multiple points of resistance, and with practices themselves, are claims with little normative substance or positive project. That is, he fails to suggest why we should oppose current power relationships or what we should replace them with. In contrast, Benner's (1990a) interpretive understanding of practices imbues them with culturally constituted meaning and the notion of communitarian good which Foucault ignored. Benner also offers an alternative to Foucault's concentration on power as essentially malevolent and coercive by proposing a different and more liberating concept of the power of caring (Benner, 1985b; 1988; 1989).

Foucault may well have countered this by suggesting that caring practices are themselves tactics of power, albeit benevolent ones. While this may be partly so, Benner's (1984) emphasis on the situational and relational importance of power grounded in an ethic of caring suggests more positive possibilities, that nurses' power can increasingly become a force for good. As Benner notes: 'The difference between empowerment and domination can be understood only if the nurse–patient relationship and the situation are understood' (Benner, 1984, p. 209).

This proposition found support in a recent hermeneutic study of the nature of nursing experience that developed Benner's work. MacLeod (1990) found that experienced ward sisters practised surveillance and observation from an involved caring stance. The situated meaning of this surveillance was not controlling and malevolent but protective and empowering. MacLeod described the sisters' observation as 'diligently watching' and 'noticing'. Diligently watching ensured that the sister could detect any potentially dangerous changes in the patient's condition while noticing enabled the sister to understand the whole situation and its salient aspects while also interpreting it.

The descriptions in Chapters 3 and 5 showed how nurses got to know the person of the parent and that their valued caring practices empowered parents. I suggest also that this research reveals an alternative to 'the gaze'. This was a concernful, involved watching-over aimed at understanding and enabling which did not overlook the other but allowed them to show up. Recall the parents' valuing of nurses who anticipated their need for information, who translated medical 'jargon', who 'took the time and trouble' to show concern and to make conversation, who created a safe and non-judgemental space within which parents could gradually take on more of their child's care and who had been with them especially during the 'black times' of their hospitalization.

The value of this watchful concern was also highlighted by the accounts given of its breakdown and absence. For example, Chapter 3's accounts from a young mother and from some of the ward nurses showed how, in this case, caring watchfulness had deteriorated into a surveillance of moral reproach and mutual suspicion. Instead of a language of caring, concern and empathic understanding there was a discourse of distrust, control and alienation.

I now move on to argue that the parents' and nurses' accounts usefully highlighted other areas of nurse caring, showing that nurses used the power of their practices to bring about transformations in the nature of their relationships with parents.

6.3.2 Parents and nurses: caring and relationships

I have tried to show how taken-for-granted ideas and concepts such as being a live-in parent and parental participation were experienced and mutually created between nurses and parents. I have argued in Chapter 5 that caring, defined as 'the alleviation of vulnerability, the promotion of growth, the preservation and extension of human possibilities in a person, a community, a family, a tradition' (Benner, 1991, p. 2) was the basis for mutually satisfying nurse–parent–child relationships. This discussion considers further the importance of nurses' caring practices in relation to resident parents' lived experiences, while broadening this understanding by also highlighting failures and breakdowns in caring.

This focus on nurse caring is important for two reasons. This study has been grounded in the interpretive phenomenological tradition where care and caring are central. For Heidegger, care is our basic way of being-in-the-world and without care, nothing matters or shows up as a concern. As Heidegger (1962, p. 274) argued: 'By working out the phenomenon of care, we have given ourselves an insight into the concrete constitution of existence'. The accounts of caring presented and interpreted can help develop an alternative perspective on caring to that proposed in recent nursing literature. In a critique of the concept of caring, Morse et al. (1990) proposed a framework which would 'clarify' caring through categorizing the research literature into various perspectives. These were caring as a human trait, as a moral ideal, as an affect, as the nurse–patient relationship and as a therapeutic intervention.

(a) Caring as a human trait?

The parents' accounts in this study gave some support to the view that caring may be a 'human trait'. Parents often spoke of caring as being a personal and often exceptional quality, something that made particular nurses 'special'. It would have been surprising if a parent had described a nurse's caring in terms of their way of being-in-the-world. However, parents alluded to Heideggerian concepts of authenticity and inauthenticity in their descriptions of nurses. They explained how some nurses seemed genuinely caring as opposed to others who seemed less sincere or who were felt to be just 'going through the motions'.

Chapter 4 showed how parents also spoke positively of nurses who did not 'take over' from them and who did not engender within them a sense of exclusion and alienation from their child's care. In this respect Heidegger (1962) warned against a solicitude which 'leaps in' for others and takes over: 'It [solicitude] can, as it were, take away "care" from the Other and put itself in his position in concern: it can leap in for him. This kind of solicitude takes over for the Other that with which he is to concern himself. The Other is thus thrown out of his own position' (Heidegger, 1962, p. 158).

He also described a solicitude, or care, which 'leaps ahead' to empower and authentically return care to the person. Parents valued nurses who created opportunities for them to be live-in parents with their child in ways which fostered involvement rather than exclusion and created possibilities rather than dependency. In describing caring, not as a trait, but as the most basic mode of being-in-the-world Benner and Wrubel (1989, p. 1) explain that 'caring . . . means that persons, events, projects, and things matter to people'. A common theme within parents' accounts of when they believed that caring was poor or absent was shown above. This was where they felt that nobody 'really cared' about them or their child, that they didn't matter to anyone. This was apparent in parents' descriptions of when they felt ignored, patronized, domineered over, alienated, excluded or not understood. Conversely, where a positive caring relationship was established, parents felt that they were as central as their child, that they too mattered. As one mother remarked, 'I don't feel I'm just there and nobody cares about me . . . I feel I'm part of the whole set-up' (17, p. 84).

(b) Caring as a moral imperative or ideal?

Theorists such as Gadow (1985; 1990) and Watson (1988a) have argued that caring is fundamentally a moral imperative. For Watson, 'caring calls for a philosophy of moral commitment toward protecting human dignity and preserving humanity' (Watson, 1988a, p. 31). She also suggests that 'caring is the moral ideal of nursing' (Watson, 1988a, p. 29). While avoiding the traditional language of moral discourse based upon rationality and principles, Benner (1990a) also argued that caring and, more specifically, a caring practice has an inalienable 'notion of good'.

The 'moral imperative' conceptualization of caring seems to suggest that caring must be a constant or given, uninfluenced by factors such as, in this case, the parent and child, the nurse or the situation. However, the accounts of both parents and nurses suggested strongly that this was not the case.

Nurses described the difficulty that they experienced in caring where they found the parent difficult to care for, or where they truly disliked the parent. This finding supports the work of Khan and Steeves (1988) who noted that while nurses believed that they **should** care for all patients equally and unconditionally, they were often unable to achieve this moral ideal. This was particularly so where they were unable to 'like' the patient and where a more 'friendly' relationship could not develop.

The nurses in the present study described wanting to care, and indeed trying to care for parents whom they believed to be difficult for particular reasons.

There were several possible outcomes here. The nurse could 'go through the motions' by being inauthentically pleasant, performing mere physical or communication 'techniques' as opposed to caring practices. The nurse may also have tried to avoid contact with the parent as much as possible. However, as I have shown, the nurse could also get beyond initial dislike and eventually develop a more caring relationship with a parent whom they may have disliked initially.

The nurses described other factors that they believed impeded caring. Temporality was important in that it was difficult for the nurses to develop a caring relationship with parents whose child was perhaps only in hospital for a very short time, for example for day surgery. The nurses recognized that such parents could still be very anxious and concerned despite the 'minor' nature of their day-surgery, yet it seemed that only the most perfunctory of relationships could be established. Temporality cannot however be considered as simple linear time whereby the longer a parent lived-in, the better the relationship. This was explained by the nurses who described how relationships could deteriorate when parents had been 'in too long'.

The position that caring is a moral imperative has a strong appeal in that most nurses say that why they became nurses was to help people or to do good in a specific way (Roach, 1987). There is, though, a danger inherent in Watson's (1988a; b) advocacy of caring as a moral ideal and that is that caring may be viewed as a purely abstract and unattainable ideal. In a commentary on Khan and Steeves's (1988) finding that nurses' caring was influenced by whether they 'liked' patients or not, Watson (1988b, p. 220) argued: 'As this work revealed, at the surface level, caring is affected perhaps by such human characteristics as liking however at the **timeless moral and philosophical level** for the profession, caring has nothing to do with liking or disliking a patient.' [My emphasis.]

There are two difficulties within this position. To argue that liking or disliking patients, or in this case parents, is somehow illegitimate is to ignore a universal human activity which cannot be wished away by appeals to a 'timeless moral and philosophical level'. Recall here the nurse who described how she formed initial impressions of parents, saying that 'We can't help doing it, we're only human'.

I suggest that the 'moral ideal', understanding, may promote a dualistic way of considering caring that suggests that there is a higher level of 'ideal' nurse caring that remains untouched by actual nursing practice and where degrees of liking do not exist. Such a position seems likely to reinforce the perceived gap between theory and practice and may also discourage examination of caring and non-caring encounters at the 'surface level' where significant improvements could be made.

(c) Caring as the nurse–parent relationship?

Several nurse theorists have described caring as being a reciprocal process between nurse and patient characterized by co-participation, dialogue and mutuality

(Benner and Wrubel, 1989; Knowlden, 1991; Green-Hernandez, 1991; Bishop and Scudder, 1990; 1991).

Chapter 5 showed that both parents and nurses valued a relationship that transcended an impersonal professional–client basis and developed into more of a friendship. The idea of friendship between nurses and in this case parents is controversial. Poslusny (1991, p. 170) argued that 'a paradigm of friendship was logically congruent with the philosophic traditions, ethics, and science of nursing'. Hunt (1991), however, contended that professional–client relations were not the same as friendship relations. In her study of symptom control team nurses she suggested that 'none of the characteristics of "friendship" can be distinguished in [their] communications' (Hunt, 1991, p. 936). Hunt (1991) also argued that proposing friendship as an aim of nurse–client relations was idealized and unrealistic if nurses were to be able to carry out distinctly professional functions.

The parents and nurses in Chapter 5 who described how 'special relationships' were formed gave support to the idea that friendship is indeed an appropriate way to characterize the close, caring relationship that developed. Both parents and nurses repeatedly described how relationships could become 'more friendly' and how the nurses or parents could become more 'like friends'. Hunt (1991) cited Skidmore (1986) in support of her contention that being friendly was not the same as being friends, because being friendly was more superficial than being friends. She also claimed that essential features of friendships are that they are reciprocal, interdependent, equitable, voluntarily chosen and based upon compatibility. Participants' accounts supported the distinction between being friendly and being a friend, but not that friendships are idealistically unachievable. The notion of authenticity is pertinent again here as parents distinguished between nurses who were being 'nice' or 'friendly' perhaps because they felt that this was their job or was expected of them. However, these were not the nurses that parents described as being friends or those with whom they had a 'special relationship'.

In relationships characterized by nurses and parents as those where they were friends, there was both reciprocity and interdependence. Participants valued relationships where there was 'come-and-go' or 'give-and-take'. Nurses and parents also described interdependent relationships, where they explained that they might not have managed without each other. It seemed also that friends, either nurses or parents, could be voluntarily chosen. Parents described how they actively sought contact with 'friendly faces', nurses who seemed to them to be most approachable and caring, or with whom they had 'hit it off' or 'just clicked'.

Conversely they described how they avoided contact with nurses whom they disliked for one reason or another. This process may not have been so explicitly followed by nurses but it seemed that there was at least an element of this voluntary choosing present, for example in the case of the staff nurse in Chapter 3 who chose to befriend and be the contact person for a 'difficult' young mother in the ward.

There was congruence between the nurses' and parents' descriptions of friendship relations and the characteristics of friendship described by Skidmore (1986).
I suggest, however, that the dimensions of friendship proposed by Poslusny
(1991) have a greater resonance with the expressed experiences of the participants
in this study. Poslusny (1991, p. 167) has proposed that 'friendship is an experience shared by individuals that creates a climate of discovery, encourages learning about oneself and others, and creates shared meaning about the world and
reality. Friendship involves discovery, learning, and sharing or meeting, engaging,
and connecting'.

Nurses whose caring practices promoted the development of friendship relations helped parents to feel that someone 'really understood' and shared in their
situation. These nurses also helped parents discover strengths and abilities that
would help them through this traumatic period. Through careful and sensitive
explanation and by being there for parents whenever they wanted to talk, these
nurses helped minimize any discrepant perspectives which parents may have
held. Their 'connected' interpersonal relationships were caring.

6.3.3 Caring as a fusion of concerns

The critique of recent caring literature by Morse *et al.* (1990) provided a useful
framework within which these findings have been further explored. However,
the assumptions underlying many of these researchers' review are themselves
questionable.

The conceptualization of caring attempted by Morse *et al.* (1990) owes more
to a tradition of thinking and scholarship which is dualistic and fragmentary
in its approach. The authors seek to establish clear distinctions between caring
and caring practices, between caring for and caring about, between the carer and
the cared for and between the process and outcomes of caring. Although
the authors do not suggest that their categories of caring are 'rigid' or 'value
judgements', there is an implicit assumption that whatever caring 'really is' must
fall primarily within one of these categories, albeit with links to others. The
authors also suggest that nursing requires a consensus view of caring which
'encompasses all aspects of nursing'. However such a strategy seems more likely
to produce a context-stripped list of 'caring behaviours' that could never be completed and which would create the illusion that if such behaviours were to be
'implemented', that this would constitute and be perceived as caring.

This study supports an alternative conceptualization of caring which stresses
not dualism but unity, not fragmentation but connectedness, not opposi-
tion but relation. It is difficult to consider Morse *et al.*'s categories without
noting the inadequacy of the descriptive and explanatory power of each of these
as they stand alone. Caring has a moral basis in that a notion of good is clearly
embedded within it. There is a sense of a moral imperative in that nurses
want to care for people and believe that this is central to nursing. Caring has an
affective component although it cannot be limited to simply an emotional

response. Caring is clearly important if positively valued interpersonal relationships are to be developed between parents and nurses. Caring is also a therapeutic intervention in that parents believed that they benefited from caring relationships.

By dissolving the distinction between subject and object, between carer and cared for, between nurse and parent, we can begin to see caring as a more mutual and co-created phenomenon. A phenomenological perspective allows caring to be viewed, not as something which nurses possess and which they 'give' to parents, nor as a private, subjective perception which parents have of something that they received. Caring instead becomes a fusion of concerns shared by nurse and parent, located in their world of common meanings and practices. The author Robert Pirsig has expressed this idea best in his allegorical novel of a father and son's motorcycle journey. He wrote that:

> The material and the craftsman's thoughts change together in a progression of smooth, even changes until his mind is at rest at the exact instant the material is right. . . . The mechanic I'm talking about doesn't make this separation. One says of him that he's 'interested' in what he's doing, that he's 'involved' in his work. What produces this involvement is, at the cutting edge of consciousness, an absence of any sense of separateness of subject and object. . . . When one isn't dominated by feelings of separateness from what he's working on, then one can be said to 'care' about what he's doing. (Pirsig, 1974, p. 289–290)

Such an understanding of caring has several implications for future research. Caring may not be best studied by abstracting it from the relationships and practice context where it occurs. In this respect, Morse *et al.*'s (1990) call for greater and more detailed categorization and definition seems a misguided quest which would quickly reach the limits of formal model-building. Such a call also ignores the differences between a behaviour and a caring practice (Benner, 1990a). This difference is crucial since it is central to the idea of a caring practice that such actions or interventions can only be interpreted to be caring within a specific local context.

I can illustrate these points through a further specific example. The nurses often described how they believed it to be extremely important to encourage parents to participate as much as possible in their child's care. However, it will be remembered that there were parents who described how, at particular times during their stay, they simply could not participate in even the most seemingly simple of child care tasks, such as changing or feeding their baby.

'Encouraging parental participation' cannot therefore be proposed or prescribed as a context-free caring behaviour or 'written standard' without regard for the particular, local and specific situation of the nurse–parent encounter. This does not mean, however, that caring is completely mystical or beyond our understanding. Caring and caring practices can be uncovered, described, interpreted and discussed as they have been here.

6.4 IMPLICATIONS

The end of all our exploring
Will be to arrive where we started
And know the place for the first time.
T.S. Eliot, 'Little Gidding'

At the outset of this study I believed that it should end with a series of specific recommendations for practitioners, managers, educators and researchers. This, I was confident, would ensure that I had answered the 'so what?' question which Strong (1979a) suggested could follow many qualitative studies which focused in detail on a small aspect of wider society. However, it is impossible to be influenced by such authors as Van Manen, Silverman, Pirsig, Benner and Heidegger, and still accept logical positivist notions of the nature of knowledge, understanding, research and practice.

Some conceptions of the role of research perpetuate a dualistic model of understanding and knowledge when they suggest that research knowledge and theory is a static entity that can be 'given' to practitioners to 'use' in their practice. Another problem inherent in the traditional perspective of knowledge as being possessed and passed on by experts is that it may subtly de-skill those whom it is ostensibly designed to benefit. I suggest that nurses have been led to see progress, knowledge, improvements, developments and expertise as being largely external to themselves and to their practice. Nurses therefore look to academia, to theory, to 'experts' for answers, thus overlooking possibilities for improvement and innovation that may exist within their own practices and their own clinical areas (Diekelmann, 1993).

My reluctance to provide pat answers to the 'problems' of live-in parents and paediatric nurses stems also from the nature of this research approach. Interpretive phenomenology is appropriate where the aim is to deepen understanding by uncovering, illuminating and interpreting important themes. It cannot describe an objective, universal reality, or discover generalizable facts about a particular situation. For these reasons, providing a list of prescriptive recommendations aimed at reforming services would be inappropriate. Has this study then been of purely academic and personal interest and of no theoretical or practical relevance to those interested and involved in paediatrics and paediatric nursing? I do not believe so.

Is this study atheoretical or anti-theory? To answer this question it is necessary to restate that interpretive or human science theory is fundamentally different from hypothetico-deductive theory. The latter has been described by Meleis (1991, p. 181) who stated that 'the aim of nursing science is to develop explanatory and prescriptive theories to understand, anticipate and control phenomena, events and situations related directly or indirectly to nursing care.' By Meleis's criteria, this study would be theoretically inadequate since there has been an explicit disavowal of explanation (in propositional or causal terms), prediction and control in relation to human caring relationships. Fortunately, within nursing there has been an increasing acceptance of the need to explore other approaches to theory that are based upon a less mechanistic, prescriptive and causal view. This view is expressed succinctly by Benner and Wrubel (1989, p. 20) who noted that 'theory about human issues and concerns must be descriptive and interpretive. Understanding is the goal.'

Within such a theoretical approach I have attempted to uncover a wide range of concerns related to the lived experiences of both parents and nurses that have often previously remained invisible, poorly understood and taken-for-granted. In my interpretive analysis I have sought to construct an account that neither merely reproduced participants' experiences nor trivialized them by superimposing a dominant or authoritative view of what they 'really meant'. The theoretical value of this research rests upon its plausibility and upon whether it has opened up possibilities. As Bleicher (1982, p. 142) noted: 'If socio-hermeneutic theory is a "reading", then it cannot be verified or falsified but only clarified (. . .) interpretations proffered cannot be judged in reference to a reality "out there" but only in relation to their fruitfulness, i.e. their potential for opening-up new ways of seeing and thereby initiating new practices.'

This does not mean, I hope, that I have performed what Wolcott (1990, p. 59) has called a 'typical academic cop-out'. Nursing is fundamentally a practice and I propose that there is much in this study that may be of considerable practical value.

Commonly invoked but little understood concepts such as family-centred care, parental participation, good and bad parents and nurse caring have been explored in depth and from a perspective that seeks to avoid the dualistic assumptions of ideal and real practice where real is almost inevitably deficient.

This research has shown that parental living-in and participation creates a series of complex and taxing demands for both parents and staff. If anyone were to imagine that having more parents living-in and 'helping out' meant that nurses had 'less to do', this study should scotch such a dangerous myth. I suggest that the involvement and commitment required by nurses to make family-centred care the meaningful advance that it promised to be, far exceeds the demands of giving purely technical or task-centred paediatric nursing care.

The study contains rich descriptions and interpretive propositions which nurses and parents may recognize and use as a basis for more mutual understanding. The study has also developed ideas that further our understandings of being a parent, the conceptualization of family, power and surveillance and the nature of the nurse–parent relationship. The study offers paediatric nurses telling accounts and insights into the lived experiences of resident parents and into the practice of paediatric nursing itself. Such accounts and insights can raise nurses' consciousness and awareness of the possibilities within their own practices, possibilities that can be taken up in order that they may create their own vision and version of more excellent paediatric family care.

I suggest that the focus of this change should be on developing nurses' understandings of resident parents and of their own nursing practices from a more phenomenological and ontological perspective. Although this may seem an abstract and distant notion to many practising nurses, educators and service managers, I believe that many of the study approaches and insights could be used as a basis for this change.

Such a movement away from a technological or instrumental understanding of live-in parents and paediatric nursing would allow nurses to gain a more meaningful appreciation of live-in parents' experiences. In view of the importance for parents of caring and feeling cared for, such a shift in focus could also allow nurses' caring practices to be more readily described and discussed. It will however be difficult, within the current climate of managerialism, with its almost exclusive focus on 'effectiveness and efficiency', for nurses to examine and nurture the good in their practices without having these transformed into universal prescriptions.

Throughout this research, dialogical understanding, mutuality and co-creation of social phenomena have been emphasized. I do not suggest for a moment that these are panaceas or that they should be the only bases of new developments, but these ways of seeing and thinking about nursing are promising future directions which paediatric nursing could pursue. There are already encouraging signs within nursing theory (Paterson and Zderad, 1988; Bishop and Scudder, 1990) and particularly within nurse education, that such ways of thinking are being developed (Bevis and Watson, 1989; Leininger and Watson, 1990; National League for Nursing, 1989; 1990; 1991). For this emphasis to carry forward, this research needs to become part of an ongoing dialogue within paediatric nursing at both ward and higher 'policy levels' that should include both nurses and parents.

Mention has previously been made of Gadamer's (1975) notion of a 'fusion of horizons' and Heidegger's (1962) conception of the 'hermeneutic circle'. I have tried to retain the sense of openness to possibilities which such a hermeneutic demands. This suggests that the most fruitful approach for the researcher who wishes to help 'implement the findings' of a study is through a continuing open dialogue with those concerned.

This study offers further support for such a dialogical rather than didactic approach to understanding the perceptions and experiences of both parents and nurses. This was brought home to me during the experiences of both the individual and Focus Group interviews. I believe that these interviews offered nurses and parents an opportunity to discuss important issues and concerns in a way that was not normally available to them. During these interviews or conversations, parents were able to discuss aspects of their lived experience which for some, could not be properly raised in any other area of discourse with professionals. They were also able to share concerns and reflect on experiences with other parents in the small Focus Groups. Similarly, the nurses were able to discuss their understandings of nursing and their everyday practices as part of a discourse where these were recognized, acknowledged and described as opposed to being judged as trivial or deficient.

It would be invaluable if service managers and practitioners were to create comfortable spaces and places for such dialogues to take place. Much is currently made in nursing of the need for 'reflective practice', although I suspect that the rhetoric of reflection far exceeds the help or time given to nurses in order that their reflection be both purposeful and meaningful. There is a clear need for nurses to become involved in dialogue, both with parents and with each other, about their everyday practices and interactions with live-in parents. Initially, nurses may feel more comfortable with informal discussion, but for nursing practices to become 'public' and part of a shared, developing nursing tradition, practitioners need to be able to write their stories or narratives. Narrative approaches to understanding nursing practice and nurse–patient relationships are becoming increasingly widely used within both practice and education (Tofias, 1989; Darbyshire, 1991; 1992). The use of these approaches within paediatrics could help nurses uncover, articulate and understand much of what this study has found to be 'unspoken'.

Paediatric nursing will be found not in lists of professional attributes or skills but in the evolving stories of nurses' everyday and taken-for-granted practices.

For myself, and possibly for the study participants, our interviews and discussions revealed other horizons and suggested alternative possibilities. Gadamer (1975, p. 269) has defined a person's horizon as 'the range of vision that includes everything that can be seen from a particular vantage point'. If this study has afforded a wider vision or offered a different vantage point, it will become a useful starting point for both parents and paediatric nurses who seek to create paediatric care that is based on excellent caring and a deeper mutual understanding.

Although there have undoubtedly been significant advances in paediatric nursing care in recent years (see, e.g., Glasper and Tucker, 1993) we do need to think differently about the parents of a hospitalized child. We need to move beyond an instrumental notion of parents as simply 'helpers' or 'performers of tasks' and of parenting as being a series of discrete child-care activities. We need instead to consider being a parent as a unique way of being in the world with a child. We need the humility to listen to parents before we plan services for them. We need to learn from them before we presume to teach them. For only from a basis of such shared understandings can a system of genuinely shared and humane care evolve.

<table>
<tr><td>

7

</td><td>

The research approach and methods

</td></tr>
</table>

7.1 THE PURPOSE AND FOCUS OF THE STUDY

In Chapter 1, I discussed the attempts that have been made to humanize paediatric hospitals by encouraging parents to live-in and to become more involved in their child's care. However, such attempts have not been matched by research which examines parents' lived experience of staying in hospital with their child. Nor has sufficient attention been paid to the experiences of paediatric nurses who are in the most direct contact with resident parents. Here, I sought to provide an interpretive account and understanding of resident parents' and paediatric nurses' lived experiences.

7.1.1 The purpose of the study

The broad purposes of this study were threefold. I sought to examine the lived experiences of parents who decided to live-in with their child during a period of hospitalization. Lived experience is understood as being the ways in which people encounter situations in relation to their interests, purposes, personal concerns and background understandings (Benner, 1985a). A similar understanding was also sought of the understandings and experiences of paediatric nurses as these related to resident parents. Finally, I wished to explore the relationships that existed between these groups. This broad purpose subsumed more specific areas that, from readings of the literature and from my professional experience, I judged to be of possible interest and importance. These included such questions as the following.

- What is the meaning for parents of being a 'live-in' parent in a paediatric ward?
- How do parents deal with the experience of being a resident mother or father?
- How do parents experience their relationships with nurses and *vice versa*?

- How do nurses experience working with parents who are living-in with their child?
- How do parents and nurses understand and operate currently popular concepts such as 'family-centred care' and 'parental involvement'?

The aim was to create a detailed and faithful interpretive account of parents' and nurses' lived experiences that would enable a better understanding of paediatric hospitalization.

7.1.2 Research approach and methods

A frequent criticism of qualitative research studies has been that researchers do not devote sufficient attention to making explicit the theoretical assumptions that underpin their research strategies (Guba, 1981; Athens, 1984; Sandelowski, 1986). However, such concerns should extend beyond questions of data collection strategies and techniques to what Giorgi (1970) terms 'approach'. This concept was defined by Giorgi thus: 'By establishing the category of "approach" we mean to take into account the researcher himself in the enterprise of science. By approach is meant the fundamental viewpoint toward man and the world that a scientist brings, or adopts, with respect to his work as a scientist, whether this viewpoint is made explicit or remains implicit' (Giorgi, 1970, p. 126).

This study was guided by a philosophy of human science which originated in the work of the early German philosopher Wilhelm Dilthey who proposed the approach of human science ('*Geisteswissenschaften*') as an alternative to prevalent natural science (Bleicher, 1980). Such a human science perspective stresses the importance of understanding the meanings that lived experience ('*Erlebnis*') have for people. This philosophy eschewed attempts to manipulate, control or objectify 'research subjects', and has had a wide appeal within the various threads of qualitative research that have developed in nursing. The selection of research methods is, however, more problematic than being guided by a particular school of thought and merits more detailed discussion. This is best illustrated through an examination of my initial difficulty in deciding upon the focus or the 'type' of research that this was to be and by pursuing and delineating the theoretical assumptions which underpinned and influenced all aspects of the method, design and interpretation.

7.1.3 The focus of the study

In a theoretical position paper, Brink and Wood (1983) posited the existence of three levels of research, graduating from Level I exploratory-descriptive, through Level II survey design, to level III experimental. In the positivist tradition Brink and Wood justified this hierarchy by stating that, as knowledge and theory regarding a particular topic evolve, then research approaches would 'progress' to the 'higher levels' described. In the early stages of deciding upon the aims of the research I found it difficult to precisely allocate any one of these pre-specified categories. In this respect MacIntyre's (1979) discussion of the similar problem that she experienced was instructive. I intended the study to be exploratory in that I wished to examine issues germane to the lived experiences of resident parents and paediatric nurses that had been previously neglected. I also wished the study to be descriptive as I proposed to seek from parents and nurses rich and detailed descriptions that would articulate the nature of their respective experiences. This, I believed, would open up the possibility of developing clearer understandings of this aspect of paediatric hospitalization. However, being mindful of Smith's caution that described or observed events do not 'speak for themselves' (Smith, 1980, p. 389), it was important that an interpretive approach be employed in order that a coherence could be brought to the data. The difficulty experienced in trying to find a mutually exclusive label that would describe an appropriate mode or level may, as MacIntyre (1979, p. 758) suggested of her own work, have reflected 'a lack of rigour and sloppiness in my approach to the research aims'. An alternative explanation proposed by MacIntyre (1979) was that such categories of research were 'more fluid' than was conventionally assumed and that elements of each may be present in a single study. A further explanation was that the initial uncertainty regarding the 'type' of study was an indication of my developing thinking in relation to qualitative and interpretive methods. I increasingly believed that some qualitative research strategies could legitimately be synthesized in a more eclectic approach.

7.1.4 The selection of a qualitative design

The research methods that I chose emerged from three main areas. Like many paediatric nurses I was aware that the relationship that existed between parents and nurses could be both satisfying and rewarding but also, on occasions, tense and uncomfortable. While working as a paediatric nurse tutor, these concerns were heightened as I realized the extent of parents' invisibility within the nursing curriculum. My feeling, which was supported through discussions with students, was that parents' experiences and concerns were treated in an almost cursory manner. As nursing professed a philosophy that valued the importance of the individual and the primacy of the individual's understandings and meanings of given situations (e.g. Paterson and Zderad, 1976; Watson, 1985), it seemed imperative that such a philosophy be recognized in the research approach. It also became apparent that such fundamental questions as my world view of the person and reality would influence the way in which I approached the research design. This world view, comprising assumptions concerning the nature of the person, reality, values, knowledge and nursing, influenced the adoption of a congruent research approach. Morgan described this more comprehensive view of the research process as 'involving choice between modes of engagement entailing different relationships between theory and method, concept and object, and researcher and researched, rather than simply a choice about method alone' (Morgan, 1983, p. 19–20).

A final reason supporting an interpretive approach related to the nature of the research questions being asked. I sought to explore areas of paediatric care that had historically been largely overlooked. I also had a 'vague hunch' that concepts such as family-centred care and parent participation were more problematic and meaning-laden than I could presently articulate. I also believed that it was important for nurses to try to gain a better understanding of the lived experiences of those whom they cared for and worked with and supported Kasch's claim that 'the ability to interpretively assess the perspectives of others appears to be an essential component of competent nursing action' (Kasch, 1986, p. 228).

7.2 THEORETICAL UNDERPINNINGS OF THE STUDY

The case for qualitative research approaches has already been convincingly demonstrated, not only in social science in general but in nursing in particular. Advances in interpretive research have built upon the seminal works of the early humanistic nursing theorists, for example, Travelbee (1971), who stressed the importance of grounding nursing within a 'human-to-human relationship' and Paterson and Zderad (1976), who were first to use an existential–phenomenological approach. These early attempts to shift nursing's world view from a dominant logical–positivist position to a more humanistic and naturalistic one have been built upon by later theorists such as Leininger (1978), Watson (1979), Parse (1981) and Benner (1984), each of whom has developed an interpretive perspective on nursing but from different philosophical origins. The question for nurse researchers is no longer 'should qualitative methods be used?' but 'When, and how best should they be used?'

7.2.1 The combining of complementary approaches

In claiming that researchers need no longer argue for the legitimacy of qualitative and interpretive methods I stress that this does not release the researcher from the obligation to explain the methods used to obtain and interpret the research data. Two qualitative approaches were used initially: grounded theory and phenomenology. While the issue of triangulation in relation to the mixing of qualitative and quantitative methods has received considerable attention (Jick, 1979; Fielding and Fielding, 1986; Mitchell, 1986), less attention has been devoted to the issues involved in using multiple qualitative theoretical approaches within a single study. The use of the combination of these two approaches arose not from any masochistic urge to make this an even more problematic endeavour, or from a desire for mere novelty. I believed, particularly at the outset, that each perspective could strengthen and improve the study in particular ways. Phenomenology, as both a philosophical orientation and method, was valuable for its focus upon describing participants' lived-experience, while grounded theory's particular methods seemed particularly capable of illuminating interaction and social relationships. A review of the nursing research literature carried out prior to data collection uncovered only one study where the researcher explicitly addressed their use of multiple theoretical approaches within the qualitative paradigm. Here Swanson-Kauffman described her approach as being 'a somewhat unique blending of the phenomenological, grounded theory and ethnographic methodologies' (Swanson-Kauffman, 1986, p. 59). She elaborated on this by explaining:

> I call this methodology 'combined' because of the different qualitative strategies that I employed to support my plan. Phenomenology as described by Giorgi, Marton and Svensson, and Oiler lent a goal to the study: to describe the human experience of miscarriage as it is lived. Spradley's ethnographic sequence provided direction for data collection. Grounded theory as described by Glaser and Strauss and clarified by Stern suggested a means for data analysis. (Swanson-Kauffman, 1986, p. 61)

I shared Swanson-Kauffman's belief that different qualitative approaches had particular strengths that could be usefully combined to gain a more complete understanding. I was concerned, however, that this approach to combining qualitative approaches seemed to be more of a 'pick 'n' mix' pragmatism than a carefully considered research strategy. For example, it seemed philosophically careless to use grounded theory only as a method of data handling without examining its philosophical basis. At the commencement, however, the benefits of combining a phenomenological and grounded theory seemed to outweigh what then seemed to be relatively trivial misgivings.

7.2.2 Phenomenology

As one of the study aims was to obtain richly detailed accounts of the lived experiences of live-in parents, phenomenology seemed the most apposite approach for, as Giorgi (1975) has stated, 'the task of the [phenomenological] researcher is to let the world of the describer, or more concretely, the situation as it exists for the subject, reveal itself through description. (...) Thus it is the meaning of the situation as it exists for the subject that descriptions yield' (Giorgi, 1975, p. 74).

This central purpose of phenomenology, the description of the lived experience of people, obtained from their own perspective, transcends many of the divergences that exist within the various schools of phenomenological thought (see Spiegelberg, 1982; Cohen, 1987; Reeder, 1987). A notable exception here is Heideggerian hermeneutic phenomenology (see Benner, 1985a; 1990b; Allen et al., 1986) which eschews the focus on individuals' subjective realities. Heideggerian phenomenology seeks to overcome the dualistic dichotomy between the subjective and objective. It rejects the idea of the person as private, and disconnected, standing over and merely responding to an objective world (Benner, 1985a). A Heideggerian hermeneutic interpretation focuses on the person in context, on commonalties of language, practices, everyday shared understandings and ontological questions concerning persons' being-in-the-world. Phenomenology is most appropriate for the study of concepts and issues within nursing whose meanings have remained unclear or unexplored (Munhall and Oiler, 1986). Phenomenological approaches have been increasingly used by nurse researchers to explore people's meanings and understandings of events and experiences in a variety of health care contexts (e.g. Field, 1981; Reimen, 1982; Drew, 1986).

7.2.3 Grounded theory

In addition to describing the lived experiences of parents, the other purpose of the study was to examine the nature of the relationships that existed and developed between paediatric nurses and live-in parents. While phenomenology's concerns seemed more expressly individualistic (although not exclusively so), grounded theory, with its origins in symbolic interactionism, appeared to be an approach that would more specifically address issues of social processes, identities and shared experiences. Blumer (1969) outlined some of the tenets of this tradition, stating that 'human beings act toward things on the basis of the meanings that the things have for them. The meaning of such things is derived from, or arises out of, the social interaction that one has with one's fellows, and these meanings are handled in, and modified through, an interpretive process used by the person in dealing with the things he encounters' (Blumer, 1969, p. 2).

The interactionist position would not assume that living-in for a parent was a major crisis or a minor adjustment, but would seek to discover how the parent defines, understands, interprets and ultimately manages the situation. Grounded theory emphasizes the importance of deriving theories and explanations of social structures and processes inductively, and by basing or grounding any explanations for observed phenomena or events firmly in the data that have been collected. I also considered a particular strength of grounded theory to be that it seemed to offer more clearly explicated data management and analysis techniques. Like phenomenology, grounded theory had frequently been used by nurse researchers who had investigated a wide range of health care behaviours and professional issues. For example, Melia (1981) had studied student nurses' socialization, Hutchinson (1986) described how neonatal nurses created meaning within their units, while Stern et al. (1984) focused on women's health issues.

7.2.4 The assumptions of grounded theory and phenomenology

An immediate difficulty facing the researcher attempting to examine these underlying assumptions is that neither symbolic interactionism nor phenomenology is a homogenous entity. Each tradition has within it a diversity of different but related schools of thought. Misiak and Sexton (1973) note of phenomenology that 'the diversity of phenomenological systems today makes a single general definition of phenomenological philosophy impossible' (Misiak and Sexton, 1973, p. 3). Meltzer *et al.* (1975) and Warshay and Warshay (1987) described the development of similar differing perspectives within symbolic interactionism. Significantly for this argument, Warshay and Warshay (1987) traced an influence back to Wilhelm Dilthey, a seminal figure in the development of hermeneutic phenomenology. Bowers (1988), in a very recent account of the value of grounded theory for nursing research, argued, almost ontologically, that an interactionist view of the self transcended mere 'role theory' and observed that, when contexts or selves overlapped or merged, 'the discomfort is clearly more than uncertainty over what role to perform. It is also a question of being, who I am, as much as doing, what actions to engage in' (Bowers, 1988, p. 37).

For the symbolic interactionist, the social world is premised upon the shared meanings of persons. The world in this sense has no meaning other than that which is ascribed by people and which, of course, is capable of being constantly refined and altered. Thus the understanding of meaning is of pivotal importance. As Blumer (1969) stated, human interaction represents 'a vast interpretive process in which people, singly and collectively, guide themselves by defining the objects, events and situations they encounter' (Blumer, 1969, p. 132).

Turning now to phenomenology's assumptions regarding these issues, I concentrate upon the strands of phenomenology that have influenced my research approach. Although influenced by earlier phenomenologists such as Dilthey, Kierkegaard and Husserl, Heidegger went on to develop a shift in philosophical questioning regarding the nature of persons and their relationship to world. In Kearney's (1986, p. 30) memorable phrase, 'he re-opened the brackets and let existence back in'.

Through his exploration of 'Being there' (*Dasein*) and its essential relatedness to our 'Being-in-the-World' (*In-der-Welt-Sein*) Heidegger (1962) shifted the focus of basic philosophical questions about the nature of persons and their relationship to the 'everydayness' of their world of existence. Rather than posing epistemological questions regarding 'What does it mean to know?' Heidegger asked what he regarded as the more fundamental question of 'What does it mean to be?' For Heidegger, persons were self-interpreting beings whose 'prime mode of access to Being' was perception in its broader existential, rather than merely sensory, meaning (Waterhouse, 1981, p. 89). It seemed therefore that strands of both phenomenology and symbolic interactionism shared certain common assumptions regarding the nature of persons and their experiences.

However, there were some discrepancies between the two perspectives, which at the outset of the research I took to be less important than the commonalities. For example; the phenomenological view of 'world' was different from the way we understand the term in common usage as being the planet, or the sum of all of the things in our immediate environment. For Heidegger and Merleau-Ponty, world, or 'lived world', was not a private sphere of existence but that which had an ontical sense, comprising all entities. World also has an ontological sense, that of a shared familiar world that makes human 'being' possible (Dreyfus, 1983). Interactionists had a different perspective on world, or 'the object world' as Blumer (1969) described it, which seemed to maintain the subjective–objective dualism that many phenomenologists sought to overcome. Research undertaken within these two theoretical perspectives must have as its prime focus the seeking of a greater understanding of the lived experiences of the participants and of the meanings that these experiences hold for them.

7.3 THE RESEARCH METHOD

It was important that the data collection methods used arose from the previously described theoretical and philosophical position. During a 10-month period of fieldwork from October, 1987 to July 1988, a total of 30 parents and 27 nurses were interviewed either individually, as a couple or in small Focus Groups. These 32 transcribed interviews, complemented by observations, conversations and occasional field notes, provided the data for interpretation.

In order to enhance the 'trustworthiness' of qualitative studies, Guba (1981) recommends that the researcher make explicit the 'decision or audit trail' in order that others may have a clear idea of the rationale behind methodological and interpretive decisions taken. Emerson (1987) made a similar case that researchers should treat the 'actual interactional and textual practices that produce ethnography (. . .) as fundamental issues worthy of their explicit, sustained attention' (Emerson, 1987, p. 77).

To address these issues I explain each aspect of the research design in more detail and acknowledge that the process of interpretation is already involved in describing the setting.

7.3.1 The setting

The fieldwork and data collection took place predominantly in two wards within a large paediatric hospital in Scotland. Ward A is a 25-bed general paediatric medical ward and Ward B is a 22-bed burns and plastic surgery unit. Ward A has a specialist interest in the care of children with diabetes mellitus and children with neurological illness and chronic neurological disorders. Ward B, in addition to caring for children who had sustained burns and scalds, also treated children who required to have 'birthmarks' removed, further plastic surgery for old burn scarring, or congenital abnormalities such as hypospadias or cleft lip and palate repaired.

I chose these two wards for several reasons. Firstly, they accommodated children with a wide variety of illnesses and injuries, thus avoiding a concentration on too narrow a group of parents and nurses as might have occurred had, for example, only an oncology unit been selected. Secondly, they provided a varied pattern of living-in among their respective resident parents, ranging from only days to weeks and even months.

The differences between these two wards had implications both for the nurses and live-in parents. Ward A's children tended to be more acutely ill with, for example, diabetic coma or suspected meningitis. Such acutely ill children tended, however, to recover relatively more quickly and in Ward A the turnover of patients was greater, with the result that live-in parents in this ward were not usually resident for as long as the parents in Ward B. In Ward B there were many children whose admissions had all of the traumatic features of an emergency. These were the children admitted with severe burns or, more commonly, with scalds. Because of the protracted nature of much of the treatment of such injuries, involving lengthy periods of waiting between skin grafts, the resident parents in Ward B tend to be in hospital for several weeks with their child.

One of the most noticeable features of both of these wards was that they were very small in relation to their present-day function of accommodating both children and parents. The lack of space was a frequently expressed complaint of both staff and parents. The introduction of open visiting also meant that 'crowd control' (Hawker, 1984; 1985) could not be regulated in the ways that it used to be, by restricting visiting hours and by strictly enforcing the number and relationship of the visitors. For example brothers, sisters, friends and relatives now visited, whereas in the past they would have been disallowed. Nurses were therefore being expected to implement a 20th-century philosophy of paediatric care in a 19th-century building.

I was familiar with this hospital, having been associated with it in different nursing capacities in the years prior to the study. This can be a double-edged sword for a researcher. Field and Morse (1985), for example, were adamant that 'the most frequent mistake that researchers make when doing participant observation is to select a setting in which they already work, or have previously worked, to conduct observations' (Field and Morse, 1985, p. 77). They added, even more ominously, that this would 'prevent the collection of valid, reliable and meaningful data.' (Field and Morse, 1985, p. 77). This, however, is an explicitly rationalist claim that data, as opposed to its analysis and interpretation, can be 'invalid' (Silverman, 1985; Smith and Heshusius, 1986). Such a claim is representative of a perspective based upon a questionable set of assumptions regarding the nature of objectivity. Field and Morse's argument is based upon the premise that there exists an objective reality or external truth which the researcher is there to discover and which can best be achieved by maintaining an objective distance. I did not share such a perspective for the reasons described earlier.

The beneficial aspects of undertaking the research in this hospital were primarily that negotiating access to the research site was made easier by the facilitative stance taken by the senior nurse managers and medical staff. My acceptance into the two chosen wards and throughout other areas of the hospital was essentially unproblematic, although I stress that I was not known to all the ward staff

7.3.2 Selecting the research participants

The selection of the study participants was a necessarily flexible process that attempted to combine the need to find participants with the expressed aim of exerting no pressure upon individuals to participate. I rejected the strategy of selecting only 'key informants' for several reasons. The very term suggests that there are other informants who may be 'non-key informants' and such a presupposition seemed contrary to an exploratory and discovery spirit. More practically, I had no way of knowing, even after familiarizing conversations, who would prove to be the 'best' informants during interviews. A further danger inherent in the key informant strategy was that 'key' might be assumed to be synonymous with articulate, extrovert or with those who seem to have the most dramatic accounts to offer (Burgess, 1984; Field and Morse, 1985). I use the term 'participant' throughout as this conveys more of the spirit in which parents and nurses shared of themselves and avoids the unfortunate 'spy' or 'betrayer' connotation which 'informant' suggests.

7.3.3 The parents

I interviewed 30 parents about their experiences of living-in with their child. These participants were 26 families: 26 mothers and four fathers. Sixteen parents participated in the focus group interviews and 14 were interviewed individually or together as a couple. The ratio of mothers to fathers reflected the fact that it was predominantly mothers who undertook to live-in with their child. Fathers have been shown to be more likely to continue with work and to care for any other children at home (Knafl and Dixon, 1984). The youngest of the mothers interviewed was 19 years old. All but two mothers were married and one mother was in the process of initiating divorce proceedings against her husband. In 16 of the families the hospitalized child was the parents' only child, while the other families were involved in making alternative arrangements for other children who were still at home. These familial factors were, as I will show, significant issues for both parents and nurses.

I decided to interview only those parents who were living-in with their child or who stayed with them for the majority of the day. This latter group of parents usually tried to be present for their child getting up in the morning and left the ward when the child had gone to sleep in the evening. The majority of the parents were sleeping in the Mothers' Unit, a small 16-bedded unit within the hospital where they would share their room with another mother. As the name suggests, this was accommodation for mothers only, although apparently fathers had been allowed to use it in very exceptional circumstances. The major difficulty here was that the rooms were twin-bedded. Three parents were staying in the social work department's Parents' Hostel, which was a short walk from the hospital and which could offer limited accommodation for mothers and fathers to share a room.

Demand for both of these facilities was heavy and not all parents who asked to live-in could be accommodated immediately. Three of the parents interviewed were sleeping beside their child's bed or in their cubicle, either through personal preference or because there was no accommodation available in the Mothers' Unit at that time. Two parents spent the majority of the day with their child but went home in the evening.

7.3.4 The children

The children were not part of this study, in that they were not interviewed or viewed as participants for research purposes. I have omitted detailed demographic or diagnostic details of children as some had been admitted with comparatively rare disorders and the possibility exists that they might be identified through these. I have, however, in the subsequent chapters, described children's particular illnesses or injuries where I believed that it was important in order to understand more fully a parent's or nurse's account of an experience.

7.3.5 The nurses

I decided to involve only qualified nurses in order to keep the scope within manageable limits and because previous studies had identified the marked influence which trained staff have in determining the overall ward 'climate' or 'atmosphere' (Pembrey, 1980; Orton, 1981; Brown, 1986). Interviews were conducted with a total of 27 qualified nurses. Twelve nurses were interviewed individually and 15 in four focus groups. Twenty-three of the nurses were paediatric-trained staff nurses at the hospital while two were RGN-trained nurses working in Ward B, undertaking the paediatric component of a Burns and Plastic Surgery course. The two other nurses were a paediatric-trained enrolled nurse and a ward sister. The nurses' experience was varied. This ranged from one nurse who had officially registered as a nurse only two weeks prior to the interview to a nurse who had 16 years' experience in various areas of paediatric nursing.

7.4 OBTAINING THE ACCOUNTS

My initial readings on the subject of qualitative and interpretative research had forewarned me that qualitative interviewing was a unique experience (Spradley, 1979; Silverman, 1985; Swanson, 1986) and quite unlike interviews with which, as a nurse and teacher, I would have been familiar, for example an admission interview or a counselling interview. I therefore carried out two 'practice interviews' prior to fieldwork. One was with a staff nurse who had left paediatrics to undergo post-registration general nurse training. The second was with a nurse who was also a former live-in parent. These 'practice runs' were valuable for several reasons. Firstly they gave me at least some experience in creating an interview that was as close as possible to everyday conversation. I also appreciated the need to tape-record such interviews carefully and with a good recorder in order that the content was both present and clearly audible.

They also demonstrated what I believe to be the necessity of personally transcribing interviews, regardless of the considerable volume of work that this created. This procedure ensured that I developed an intimate knowledge of each interview, gained from the discipline of listening attentively to every word of the tape recording during transcribing.

A final benefit that accrued from these practice interviews was that, after my fledgling attempts at qualitative data analysis, I had some ideas from the interviews that served as guiding questions, 'foreshadowed problems' (Malinowski, 1922) or 'sensitizing concepts' (Blumer, 1954). I stress, however, that these were the most general of ideas and were not allowed to set a pre-specified agenda for the actual interviews.

7.4.1 Bracketing, guiding and generative questions

Having even very general guiding questions prior to data collection is controversial within phenomenology and Husserl's concept of 'bracketing' (*epoche*) seemed the crucial issue here. Husserl (1962) wrote of the need to achieve *epoche* or the suspension of all previously held assumptions, beliefs and judgements about an issue prior to and during its investigation. Similarly, Kvale (1983, p. 176) suggested that researchers should make themselves 'presuppositionless' where they 'remain open to new and unexpected phenomena'.

What was less clearly explained was how such a denial (even temporarily) of all background knowledge and assumptions was to be achieved. This is especially problematic in view of the Heideggerian concepts of 'forehaving' and background meanings which reject such a possibility of 'presuppositionless' understanding or involvement. Grounded theory has no difficulty with the researcher's preparation of general questions and indeed encouraged the raising of initial 'generative questions' (Strauss, 1987).

In order to achieve rapprochement between these positions, I approached the interviews and fieldwork with some very general questions and wider issues that would give at least an initial focus and direction while also being prepared to let the participants take these interviews in the directions that they believed to be most important for them.

I also tried to recognize and set aside any assumptions that I might have had regarding any possible outcomes or findings that might be produced in order that I would be better able to accept and follow the directions that the participants themselves would wish to take. I have also tried to make my assumptions explicit, both in these introductory discussions and throughout the book.

7.4.2 Engaging the participants' involvement

A crucial consideration in this research was that I was expecting parents of sick and injured children to discuss, with a relative stranger, intimate details of what for most would rate as one of the most traumatic events of their lives. Similarly, as an educator and researcher, I was expecting nurses to 'go on record', albeit anonymously, with their ideas regarding some of the most personal and professionally contentious aspects of their work.

It was clear to me that if I wished parents and nurses to agree to be interviewed, then I would first have to establish a climate of trust and familiarity. The kind of dialogue that I sought could not realistically have been obtained through 'cold calling'. To create such a climate was the primary purpose of the period of fieldwork spent in the wards. This was not intended to be a period of formal participant observation in the strict ethnographic sense (Spradley, 1980). During the period of fieldwork, I was, however, able to observe live-in parents and nurses in a variety of interactions. Not all of these observations were recorded as *bona fide* fieldnotes, but any interactions or events which I thought significant were noted. These often formed the basis for a general question or probe during an interview or became a topic of conversation.

I can best describe the time that I spent in the wards as being a period of familiarization. Not only was I becoming aware of the rhythms and atmospheres of the wards but what was more important was that the parents and nurses were becoming familiar with both the study and me. I made a point of introducing myself to any new resident parents and was identified by a name badge which said 'Philip Darbyshire: Nurse Researcher'.

I had also prepared a printed handout for both parents and nurses explaining briefly, in question and answer format, who I was and what the study was about. This proved to be a useful icebreaker in my initial approaches to new parents and usually allowed me to engage in some general conversation. These initial conversations with parents were vitally important in establishing a climate of trust and relaxation without which it would have been insensitive, if not impossible, to ask parents to participate in a taped interview.

During these initial conversations I asked parents and nurses if they would object to me jotting down in my notebook any points of interest or questions that our conversation might prompt for future use in the study. As this was done deliberately casually, openly and as non-threateningly as possible, no-one objected to this and the notebook did not become the impediment to rapport that I had initially feared.

A further advantage of these familiarizing conversations was that they allowed me to establish my credibility with parents. I found it useful to imagine potential participants saying to themselves, 'Why on earth should I tell this person anything?' In this respect, the parents were usually interested (and not a little surprised) that someone should be seeking their understandings of their situation.

Another factor that helped foster trust was my explanation that I was not only a researcher but also a paediatric nurse. Far from this creating or furthering a 'them and us' divide as I had feared, it was my impression that this was a factor which reassured parents in some way and assisted rapport. Finally I mentioned that I too was a parent, although my daughter had never been admitted to hospital. I have no doubt that this helped to create a sense of 'shared parenthood' between the parents and myself.

This familiarizing and informal conversation with parents was an essential pre-requisite to asking whether the parents would agree to taking part in a tape-recorded interview. Parents seemed less apprehensive about the interviews as a result, which may have positively influenced the quality of the interviews as data. Such an approach may also have been particularly effective in helping to secure a very high 'response rate'. Only one nurse from Wards A and B chose not to participate. All of the parents who were asked to participate in an interview after initial conversations agreed.

7.4.3 The interviews

The interviews were as close to natural, informal conversation as possible. My aim was to allow the participants to take the interview in the directions that they felt to be most important and salient to them. However, as long silences can be uncomfortable in interviews, particularly for the respondents, who may feel that they are not 'performing well' or giving 'enough' or the 'right' information, I had a list of broad trigger topics derived from the practice interviews and conversation fieldnotes which I would use to give an opening for further discussion. An important point in relation to participants feeling uncomfortable concerns the use of the tape recorder in interviews. This proved to be of little or no concern to participants, none of whom asked that their interview should not be recorded.

I considered it important that the interviews be held within the hospital or ward in order to retain a sense of context. I also believed that this would help in keeping the salient aspects of the situation at the forefront of participants' thoughts. All the individual and couple interviews were held either in a vacant side room within the ward or, in some cases, in the ward's Intensive Care Unit when empty. These locations had a marked advantage over, for example, an office, as there were no external interruptions such as ringing telephones. All the focus group interviews were held around a table within the hospital's small lecture theatre, which afforded the same advantages.

I was aware that parents would be reluctant to leave their child at particular periods and for any great length of time. This made complete flexibility in relation to interviews necessary. These were fitted in when, for example, the child was having an afternoon nap and were frequently cancelled and rescheduled due to changes in a child's condition. The focus group interviews were more difficult to organize and were all held at around 10 pm as this was the only time of day when parents were able to get together, when their child had 'settled down' for the night.

Four small focus group interviews were held with different groups of parents and an equal number with different groups of nurses. Focus group interviews have their origins in marketing, advertising and consumer research (Calder, 1977; Morgan and Spanish, 1984) and have rarely been used in health care research (Beck *et al.*, 1986; Heimann-Ratain *et al.*, 1985; Festervand, 1985). Festervand explained that 'the focus group interview is a variation of the depth interview. In the focus group interview, a small number of individuals are brought together and allowed to interact rather than being interviewed one at a time, as in the depth interview' (Festervand, 1985; p. 200).

The decision to use focus group interviews was made on interpretive grounds. I had listened to parents describe the conversations that they had with each other in the Mothers' Unit or in the coffee room. They spoke of how they had supported another mother at a particularly difficult time, or had talked of some aspect of the hospital or their care that would, as one mother suggested, 'have the staff's ears burning'. Nurses, of course, had similar informal discussions where aspects of the day's work (and it must be recognized, where parents and children) were often discussed. Focus group interviews offered a way to capture some of this context of being a parent or nurse but in the security of the company of others and held the potential to enrich the initial concepts and ideas which were emerging from the individual interviews.

Parents and nurses were given a brief information handout which I also posted on each of the ward notice boards and in the Mothers' Unit and Parents' Hostel. I imagined that these would make the sessions seem informal and non-threatening, but what I had initially failed to consider was the importance of the familiarizing that had been so crucial in relation to the individual interviews.

This was brought home clearly on the night of the first scheduled parents' group interview when no-one at all attended. Consequently, I made a point of visiting the other wards within the hospital to talk briefly with resident parents and to let them know who I was and what I was doing. This seemed to work and the subsequent focus group interviews had respectively three, four, four and five parents attending.

The nurses' group interviews were less difficult to organize and took place either at the end of a shift or during the overlap of shifts when there were maximum staff present to cover for absence. During these interviews there were groups of two, three, five and five nurses. Both the individual and the focus group interviews lasted between approximately 45 minutes and two hours, the average length being around one hour.

7.4.4 Ethical considerations

Prior to the fieldwork, the medical ethics committee of the relevant Health Board was contacted and informed of the nature of the study. Formal approval to proceed was given in September 1987 prior to data collection. Permission to undertake the fieldwork was also sought from senior nurse managers at the hospital and from the ward sisters of Wards A and B. The Hospital Management Committee and the chairman of the Medical Staff Committee were also informed of the study. Each consultant involved with both of the study wards was also contacted for permission to involve parents under their care and all agreed to this.

The decision to broaden the data collection through focus group interviews with a wider group of parents was communicated to the hospital's local ethical committee representative who confirmed that this was acceptable. These were the more formal, procedural steps taken to ensure a sound ethical basis for the study but, as I suggested in relation to the previous sections, this kind of 'bare bones' information tells only half a story.

Because of its expressly non-manipulative and un-controlling stance, qualitative research runs the risk of imagining itself to be, as Dingwall (1980, p. 873) suggests, '*a priori* on the side of the angels'. This notion may have arisen from the erroneous perception that qualitative research is the voice of the 'underdog' or merely the representation of the voice of the comparatively powerless against the more powerful (see Becker, 1967). It may also be assumed that, in such studies, the barriers between researcher and 'subject' are broken down, resulting in the end of the power differential found in more positivistic approaches. With this imagined levelling of power comes an often unstated assumption that the need for ethical vigilance is commensurably diminished. However, as Foucault has shown, power 'is exercised through a net-like organization in which all are caught' (Smart, 1985, p. 79). It cannot simply be given away.

The most salient ethical issues were, I believe, those of informed consent, confidentiality, anonymity and the researcher–participant relationship. Each of these merits further discussion in constructing an explicit ethical evaluation of this study.

Informed consent is almost universally accepted as being not only a good thing but an essential prerequisite of ethical research. The qualitative researcher faces particular problems here as contact with people may occur over a lengthy period of fieldwork, necessitating not merely informed consent in the usual sense of a single signature but a continuing willingness to participate in what might be a changing research agenda.

Such consent is more processual than the final signing of the traditional consent form that may lead the researcher to conclude that such a signing obviates the need for ethical sensitivity and reflection to permeate the entire study. In practice, the steps that were taken to ensure a truly informed process consent were as follows:

- The nature of the study was discussed with all resident parents and nurses who were involved in any of the fieldwork conversations and interviews. This was supplemented with written information sheets which were given to all those involved.
- Participants were assured that the study had no covert purpose or hidden agenda, for example to evaluate nurse performance. The research purpose was made explicit as was the need to collect data through conversation and interview. Notes were not written surreptitiously, but openly during discussions and conversations.
- During interviews it was made clear to participants that they could control the

interview as they wished, by declining without prejudice to discuss any topic or to answer any question which they wished not to. If, during interviews, I sensed that participants were uncomfortable with a topic I would check whether they really did wish to discuss this area or whether they would rather not. In the event, no one declined to discuss any particular topic.

Confidentiality and anonymity are equally problematic within qualitative research and raised particular dilemmas for me. Archbold (1986, p. 158) anticipated this when she noted that 'in small social systems where everyone knows everyone, even the slight cues of demographic descriptors (age, sex, number of children) may reveal a person's identity'. Archbold also cautioned that 'in some cases, it may be necessary to discard or thoroughly disguise data to protect subjects' (Archbold, 1986, p. 158). While the usual conventions of not naming the research site or participants were followed, this might be insufficient to prevent the determined reader from guessing accurately the hospital in question. There are after all, comparatively few paediatric hospitals in Scotland. Similarly, within the hospital, the amount of contextual detail that is given regarding the two wards would lead to their easy identification by anyone who knows the hospital. Steps were taken however in order to protect the confidentiality of participants. These were as follows.

- All parents and nurses were identified by a randomly allocated initial or pseudonym. Thus 'Mrs S' or 'Nurse T' in an interview excerpt would not necessarily have a surname beginning with 'S' or 'T'. The names of any family or friends mentioned have also been changed.
- All nurses are referred to only as 'nurse' regardless of their rank.
- Any children mentioned are referred to by a pseudonym and the gender of any children named has been randomly assigned and re-assigned throughout the book. Where a child had a particularly unusual illness or injury that might easily identify them I have changed this while trying to retain the essential character of the disorder. For example I did not substitute the name of a short-term acute illness for a long-term chronic illness.
- Where participants made reference to any other named parent or nurse, this particular name has been replaced by a pseudonym.
- During the transcription of the interviews, it became clear that certain people could perhaps be recognized through their use of a particular figure of speech or by the repetition of a particular phrase. In these cases the identifying phrase has been deleted or rephrased if it was thought particularly important to the meaning of the extract.
- For the purposes of this study, detailed demographic information factors were of minimal importance and hence have been omitted in order to further protect the participants' anonymity.

While these strategies helped to ensure confidentiality for the participants, they also ensured their anonymity. It may seem paradoxical, but for interpretive research that seeks to uncover and describe lived experience, this anonymity must also be considered to be a limitation of the study. The participants have necessarily lost much of the rich personal detail that helped to make up their particular context and personhood. When their individuality is stripped away to reduce them to merely 'Mother 1', 'Father' or 'Nurse S' it is as if the person has been lost to confidentiality. I saw no way to resolve this dilemma that would have ensured both confidentiality and a fuller personal biography and therefore accepted this as a necessary, if unfortunate, trade-off that must be made in research.

The importance of the relationship between the researcher and the participants has been recognized as being of paramount importance in qualitative research. At its most fundamental level, the failure to achieve or maintain good relationships with all of those involved in fieldwork will ensure that data collection is made difficult if not impossible. However such trusting, friendly relationships harboured their own ethical problems. For example, the researcher is often advised to be non-judgemental regarding the expressed views of the participants. In practice this was more problematic.

Consider the example of a nurse who was highly critical of a parent or of parents in general. Hinting at, or overtly disapproving of such attitudes might have pressured the nurse to alter or modify her expressed perspective, whereas suggesting agreement with the view in order to gain further elaboration smacks of entrapment.

This research approach also raised issues of involvement, friendships and trust between the participants and myself that extended from the earliest stages of planning to the writing and dissemination of findings. In furthering awareness of the ethical dimension of qualitative research, I support Dingwall's claim that formalized ethical codes and protocols are of minimal value. Of greater importance are the person and fieldwork practices of the researcher. As Dingwall (1980) noted: 'In the last analysis, ethical fieldwork turns on the moral sense and integrity of the researcher negotiating the social contract which leads his subjects to expose their lives' (Dingwall, 1980, p. 885).

I recognized and tried to deal with these issues during the fieldwork in several ways. Among these were:

- being genuinely interested in the participants and their respective situations and being friendly, self-disclosing and helpful where possible;
- being non-judgemental and 'allowing' participants to express what they perhaps felt were unpopular views – this was done in as neutral a way as I could manage, perhaps by saying that I understood how they could come to feel this way and moving on to ask for further clarification of their particular perspective;
- my experience as a paediatric nurse was of real value in knowing how and when to approach and converse with parents and nurses and when it would be most ethical (and tactful) to stay silent and unobtrusive.

This section has been deliberately detailed in order to move ethical thinking about research to a more prominent place in a methods discussion. I believe that merely reporting Ethics Committee decisions is an insufficient response to the particular ethical issues inherent within the qualitative or interpretative research paradigm.

7.4.5 Interpretive analysis

The more mechanical aspects of data analysis were that transcribed text was printed on to wide, tractor-feed computer paper which allowed me to leave a very wide right-hand margin where I made short code notation or more lengthy interpretive comments during the line-by-line analysis recommended by Strauss (1987). Initial interpretive readings yielded many codes, which were noted in a card index system.

Emergent categories were then questioned and contemplated more rigorously. This process of questioning the data was usefully described by Hammersley and Atkinson (1983, p. 178) as 'using the data to think with'. During this process I sought to identify themes and patterns, similarities and dissimilarities and observations, comments and events that seemed meaningful for the participants in relation to their lived experience.

A further interpretive strategy involved being constantly 'reflexive' (Hammersley and Atkinson, 1983), which involved a sustained, reflective dialogue with the data. This is implied in grounded theory's concept of the constant comparative method (Glaser and Strauss, 1967) and is also explicitly advocated in phenomenological research where the process of hyperattending to the data has been described as 'dwelling with' the data or 'intuiting' (Johnson, 1975). Similarly, within the approach of the hermeneutic circle, the analyst would not approach interpretation in a rectilinear fashion but would constantly re-evaluate and re-interpret data in order that 'the whole is understood from its parts and the parts from the whole' (Schleiermacher, 1977, p. 5–6).

Writing memos was another interpretive technique used in order that I could keep a record of how my thoughts regarding various themes and issues were developing, a sort of 'thinking aloud on paper'. Interpretive analysis of the data was an integral part of the entire research process that helped to determine the focus and direction of the study as it evolved and which was still ongoing as the study was being written.

Silverman (1989, p. 73), in a recent theoretical position paper, echoed my concerns expressed in Chapter 1 regarding studies that made 'assertions based upon no more than supportive gobbets of data'. It was important, therefore, that direct quotations from the participants' interviews were used frequently rather than sparingly, in order that the reader could better follow the interpretive analysis. This also countered any possibility that the study would render participants' accounts invisible or transform them entirely into theoretical concepts.

In keeping with the study aims, it was important that the participants' accounts were not used in order to perform mere 'ironies' (Silverman, 1985, p. 21). Thus parents' accounts were not treated as being simply one version of an external reality which could subsequently be undermined or 'disproved' by reference to the nurses' accounts or *vice versa*. This did not, of course, obviate the possibility that parents and nurses might hold discrepant perspectives regarding various phenomena.

7.4.6 Rigour and trustworthiness

Qualitative studies must address the issue of research rigour if they are to avoid the charge that 'anything goes' (Silverman, 1985). This is not to say, however, that the specific criteria devised to evaluate more positivist or quantitative work can be applied to qualitative work. As Borman *et al.* (1986, p. 42) noted: 'From this perspective, qualitative research is criticized for not being something it never intended to be, and is not given credit for its strengths'. I contend that criteria for reliability and generalizability as understood within the quantitative research tradition are inappropriate within an interpretive approach. This is a recognition not of a weakness within interpretive research but of the complexity and fluidity of social life and of the presence and effect that the researcher has upon every element of the study. Strong (1979a, p. 250) argued that the quest for 'guaranteed interpretation' is delusory and that 'the best we can hope for in this world, even if we study practical reasoning, is a plausible story'.

The specific measures taken to enhance the study's plausibility are summarized as follows. Descriptive and interpretive adequacy was sought through continuous reflexivity (Hammersley and Atkinson, 1983) which recognized the essential linkage between the social and technical process of data collection and interpretation. As expected, the early interviews were more exploratory than later ones. As I listened to the earlier interviews and read the first transcripts, themes, events, feelings, commonalities and discrepancies emerged which seemed to be of greater importance to the participants and which were then raised as more specific issues in subsequent interviews.

Familiarizing conversations took place with each participant in order that they might approach the interview with minimal apprehension and reticence. Individual and co-joint interviews were complemented by the use of focus group interviews. The 10 months of fieldwork within the wards was prolonged enough to obtain an adequate number of interviews to satisfy the aims and purpose. Frequent use has been made of directly quoted material from the participants' accounts in order to illustrate interpretive insights. Participant and researcher interpretations have also been explicitly delineated.

Respondent validation, where preliminary interpretations or later findings are presented to the participants themselves for comment and 'validation', was not undertaken. One reason for this was the logistic difficulties that would have been involved, for example in contacting and meeting with parents who had since left the ward. A more pertinent analytic reason, however, was my concurrence with Bloor (1983), who cautioned against using respondents' comments to judge the credibility of the researcher's interpretation of the situation.

Rather, such responses require to be treated as problematic and as interesting constructed responses to a social situation in their own right (Bloor, 1983; Silverman, 1985).

Developing ideas and interpretations were, however, critiqued during peer discussions with fellow research students. Towards the end and after completion of the study, findings were presented to audiences of paediatric nurses in the UK, Canada, New Zealand, USA and Australia where reactions were very positive and corroborative. Discussions here have also stimulated some re-interpretation along alternative lines of thought.

Despite these attempts to create plausible interpretations, the question remains: 'What if someone does not "see" the adequacy of our interpretation, does not accept our reading?' (Taylor, 1985b, p. 17). To this question, there is practically no answer that does not lead towards a chimerical, epistemological certainty. As Taylor explained: 'We can only convince an interlocutor if at some point he shares our understanding of the language concerned. If he does not, there is no further step to be taken in rational argument' (Taylor, 1985b, p. 18).

7.5 CONCLUDING COMMENTS

This section has been necessarily lengthy and discursive in order to provide the fullest research context within which the findings may be best understood. Even this, however, does not tell the whole story.

Accounts of published research tend to perpetuate the view that a particular method is selected at the outset and that this method is simply 'used' unproblematically and unchanged throughout the study. My experience was that, as my understandings of phenomenological approaches and philosophy developed, my approaches to the interpretive analysis shifted in focus. For example, I began to see more fundamental differences between grounded theory and phenomenology, particularly hermeneutic phenomenology, than I had appreciated at the outset. I became concerned that I was using grounded theory's approach to coding and categorizing while recognizing that my interpretive insights were drawing increasingly on Heideggerian and hermeneutic phenomenology.

This may account for my frustration as I struggled fruitlessly to find a 'Core Category' or 'Basic Social Process' that would subsume all of the rest of the data. The only way in which all of my 'codes and categories' would fit into an overarching core category was if the category were so general as to be meaningless. I also began to sense that my grounded theory strategies were fragmentary and reductionist. My thinking was being forced into the construction of analytic laws and causal mechanisms which would explain the 'reality' of the research setting rather than enabling me to dwell with the stories of the participants and enable an interpretive uncovering which would preserve context. Such analytic thinking in its search for closure, answers and ultimate clarity seemed to fail to acknowledge the circularity of understanding (Gadamer, 1975). In contrast, dwelling thinking

(Heidegger, 1966) allowed for a keeping open, an essential incompleteness in the dialogue that left a space for the important presence of the reader.

A specific example of my growing dissonance with grounded theory was my initial attempts to keep both theoretical and observational notes as suggested by Glaser and Strauss (1967) and Schatzman and Strauss (1973). This seemed a logical strategy initially, but I later questioned the philosophy underlying this strategy. It seemed that this approach assumed that there were data that were interpreted and thus deemed to be theoretical while another class of 'brute data' (Rabinow and Sullivan, 1979) were merely observational and thus presumably uninterpreted. Such an assumption seemed increasingly at odds with a central assumption of hermeneutic phenomenology, that there can be no interpretation-free 'data' since we are all self-interpreting beings who are within our pre-understandings.

These comments are intended to enhance the reflective element of the study and to highlight that its philosophical and hence methodological basis was not static over the six years of its undertaking. They are also intended to avoid glossing over or ignoring real methodological difficulties. They cannot 'invalidate' the previous sections of this chapter, as these descriptions remain accurate accounts of my earlier methodological thinking.

References

Adamson, E.F.StJ. and Hull, D. (1984) *Nursing Sick Children*, Churchill Livingstone, Edinburgh.

Agan, R.D. (1987) Intuitive knowing as a dimension of nursing. *Advances in Nursing Science*, **10**(1), 63–70.

Algren, C.L. (1985) Role perception of mothers who have hospitalised children. *Children's Health Care*, **14**(1), 6–9.

Allan, G. and Crow, G. (1989) *Home and Family: Creating the Domestic Sphere*, Macmillan, London.

Allen, D.G. (1985) Nursing research and social control: Alternative models of science that emphasise understanding and emancipation. *Image: Journal of Nursing Scholarship*, **17**(2), 58–64.

Allen, D., Benner, P. and Diekelmann, N. (1986) Three paradigms for nursing research, in *Nursing Research: Methodology; Issues and Implementations*, (ed. P. Chinn), Aspen & Co., Rockville, MD.

Anonymous (1984) One mother's view. *The Practitioner*, **228**(1396), 960.

Anstice, E. (1970) 'Nurse, where's my mummy?' *Nursing Times*, **66**(48), 1513–1518.

Arango, P. (1990) A parent's perspective: Making family centred care a reality. *Children's Health Care*, **19**(1), 57–62.

Archbold, P. (1986) Ethical issues in qualitative research, in *From Practice to Grounded Theory*, (eds W.C. Chenitz and J.M. Swanson), Addison-Wesley, Menlo Park, CA.

Armitage, S. (1980) Non-compliant recipients of health care. *Nursing Times*, **76**, 1–3.

Athens, L.H. (1984) Scientific criteria for evaluating qualitative studies. *Studies in Symbolic Interaction*, **5**, 259–268.

Baruch, G. (1981) Moral tales: Parents' stories of encounters with the health professions. *Sociology of Health and Illness*, **3**(3), 275–296.

Beardslee, W.R. and De Maso, D.R. (1982) Staff Groups in a paediatric hospital: Content and coping. *American Journal of Orthopsychiatry*, **52**, 712–718.

Beck, L., Trombetta, W. and Share, S. (1986) Using focus group sessions before decisions are made. *North Carolina Medical Journal*, **47**(2), 73–74.

Beck, M. (1973) Attitudes of parents of pediatric heart patients towards patient care units. *Nursing Research*, **22**(4), 334–338.

Becker, H. (1967) Whose side are we on? *Social Problems*, **14**, 239–248.

Beckett, J. (1986) The parents' view. *American Association for Respiratory Care Times*, **11**(6), 66, 68.

Bell, C. and Newby, H. (1977) Epilogue, in *Doing Sociological Research*, (eds C. Bell and H. Newby), Allen and Unwin, London.

Bellah, R.N., Masden, R., Sullivan, W.M. *et al.* (1985) *Habits of the Heart: Individualism and Commitment in American Life*, University of California Press, Berkeley, CA.

Benner, P. (1984) *From Novice to Expert: Excellence and Power in Clinical Nursing*, Addison-Wesley, Menlo Park, CA.

Benner, P. (1985a) Quality of life: A phenomenological perspective on explanation, prediction and understanding in nursing science. *Advances in Nursing Science*, **8**(1), 1–14.

Benner, P. (1985b) Preserving caring in an era of cost-containment, marketing and high technology. *Yale Nurse*, **August** 12–20.

Benner, P. (1988) Nursing as a caring profession. Paper presented at the American Academy of Nursing, 16–18 October, Kansas City, MO.

Benner, P. (1989) The quest for control and the possibilities of care. Paper presented at the Applied Heidegger Conference, September, Berkeley, CA.

Benner, P. (1990a) The moral dimension of caring, in *Knowledge About Care and Caring*, (eds, J.S. Stevenson and T. Tripp-Reimer), American Academy of Nursing, Kansas City, MO.

Benner, P. (1990b) Interpretive phenomenology as theory and method. Department of Physiological Nursing, University of California at San Francisco. Unpublished mimeo.

Benner, P. (1990c) The primacy of caring, the role of experience, narrative and community in skilled ethical comportment. Department of Physiological Nursing, University of California at San Francisco. Unpublished paper.

Benner, P. (1991) The role of experience, narrative and community in skilled ethical comportment. *Advances in Nursing Science*, **14**(2), 1–21.

Benner, P. and Tanner, C. (1987) How expert nurses use intuition. *American Journal of Nursing*, **87**(1), 23–31.

Benner, P. and Wrubel, J. (1989) *The Primacy of Caring: Stress and Coping in Health and Illness*, Addison-Wesley, Menlo Park, CA.

Bergum, V. (1988) *Woman to Mother: A Transformation*, Bergin & Garvey, South Hadley.

Berman, D.C. (1966) Pediatric nurses as mothers see them. *American Journal of Nursing*, **66**(11), 2429–2431.

Betz, C.L. and Poster, E.C. (1984) Incorporating play into the care of hospitalised children. *Issues in Comprehensive Pediatric Nursing*, **7**, 343–355.

Beuf, A.H. (1979) *Biting off the Bracelet: A Study of Children in Hospital*, University of Pennsylvania Press, Philadelphia, PA.

Bevis, E.O. and Watson, J. (1989) *Toward a Caring Curriculum: A New Pedagogy for Nursing*, National League for Nursing, New York.

Bishop, A.H. and Scudder, J.R.Jr (1990) *The Practical, Moral and Personal Sense of Nursing: A Phenomenological Philosophy of Practice*, State University of New York Press, New York.

Bishop, A.H. and Scudder, J.R.Jr (1991) Dialogical care and nursing practice, in *Anthology on Caring*, (ed. P. Chinn), National League for Nursing, New York.

Bleicher, J. (1980) *Hermeneutics as Method, Philosophy and Critique*, Routledge, London.

Bleicher, J. (1982) *The Hermeneutic Imagination*, Routledge, London.

Bloor, M.J. (1983) Notes on member validation, in *Contemporary Field Research: A Collection of Readings*, (ed. R.M. Emerson), Little, Brown & Co., Boston, MA.

Blumer, H. (1954) What is wrong with social theory? *American Sociological Review*, **1**, 3–10.

Blumer, H. (1969) *Symbolic Interaction: Perspective and Method*, Prentice Hall, Englewood Cliffs, NJ.

Bogdan, R., Brown, M.A. and Foster, S.B. (1982) Be honest but not cruel: Staff/parent communication on a neonatal unit. *Human Organisation*, **41**(1), 6–16.

Bollnow, O.F. (1961) Lived space. *Philosophy Today*, **5**, (1/4), 31–39.

Bordo, S. (1986) The Cartesian masculinisation of thought. *Signs*, **11**(3), 439–456.

Borman, K.M., LeCompte, M.D. and Goetz, J.P. (1986) Ethnographic and qualitative research design and why it doesn't work. *American Behavioural Scientist*, **30**(1), 42–57.

Boulton, M.G. (1983) *On Being a Mother: A Study of Women With Pre-School Children*, Tavistock Press, London.

Bowers, B.J. (1988) Grounded Theory, in *Paths to Knowledge: Innovative Research Methods for Nursing*, (ed. B. Sarter), National League for Nursing, New York.

Bowlby, J. (1953) *Child Care and the Growth of Love*, Penguin, Harmondsworth.

Brain, D.J. and MacLay, I. (1968) Controlled study of mothers and children in hospital. *British Medical Journal*, **1**, 278–280.

Brink, P.J. and Wood, M.J. (1983) *Basic Steps in Planning Nursing Research: From Question to Proposal*, Wadsworth Health Science Division, Monterey, CA.

Brossat, S. and Pinell, P. (1990) Coping with parents. *Sociology of Health and Illness*, **12** (1), 69–83.

Brown, J. and Ritchie, J.A. (1990) Nurses' perceptions of parent and nurse roles in caring for hospitalised children. *Children's Health Care*, **19**(1), 28–36.

Brown, R. (1986) The social organisation of work in two paediatric wards in relation to patient and task allocation. University of Warwick, Warwick. PhD Thesis.

Brown, R.A. (1989) *Individualised Care*. Scutari Press, London.

Brunvand, J.H. (1981) *The Vanishing Hitchhiker: Urban Legends and their Meaning*, Picador, London.

Brunvand, J.H. (1984) *The Choking Doberman and Other 'New' Urban Legends*, Penguin, Harmondsworth.

Buber, M. (1958) *I and Thou* , 2nd edn, (trans. R.G. Smith), Charles Scribner, New York.

Burgess, R.G. (1984) *In the Field: An Introduction to Field Research*, George Allen & Unwin, London.

Calder, B. (1977) Focus groups and the nature of qualitative marketing research. *Journal of Marketing Research*, **14**, 353–364.

Callery, P. and Smith, L. (1991) A study of role negotiation between nurses and the parents of hospitalised children. *Journal of Advanced Nursing*, **16**(7), 772–781.

Carpenter, S. (1980) Observations of mothers living-in on a paediatric unit. *Journal of Maternal and Child Health*, **October**, 368-373.

Chopoorian, T. (1986) Reconceptualising the environment, in *New Approaches to Theory Development*, (ed. P. Moccia), National League for Nursing, New York.

Cleary, J. (1977) The distribution of nursing attention in a children's ward. *Nursing Times (Occasional Paper)*,**73**(28), 93–96.

Cleary, J. (1979) Demands and responses: The effects of the style of work allocation on the distribution of nursing attention, in *Beyond Separation: Further Studies of Children in Hospital*, (eds D.J. Hall and M. Stacey), Routledge & Kegan Paul, London.

Cleary, J., Gray, O.P., Hall, D.J. *et al.* (1986) Parental involvement in the lives of children in hospital. *Archives of Disease in Childhood*, **61**(8), 779–787.

Cohen, M.Z. (1987) A historical overview of the phenomenological movement. *Image: Journal of Nursing Scholarship*, **19**(1), 31–34.

Consumers Association (1980) *Children in Hospital: A Which? Campaign Report*, Consumers Association, London.

Coucovanis, J.A. and Solomons, H.C. (1983) Handling complicated visitation problems of hospitalized children. *American Journal of Maternal-Child Nursing*, **8**(2), 131–134.

Craik, J. (1989) The making of mother: The role of the kitchen in the home, in *Home and Family: Creating the Domestic Sphere*, (eds G. Allan and G. Crow), Macmillan, London.

Darbyshire, P. (1991) Nursing reflections. *Nursing Times*, **87**(36), 27–28.

Darbyshire, P. (1992) Telling stories, telling moments. *Nursing Times*, **88**(1), 22–24.

Davis, B. (1984) What is the nurse's perception of the patient? in *Understanding Nurses: The Social Psychology of Nurses*, (ed. S. Skevington), John Wiley & Sons, Chichester.

Davis, F. (1963) *Passage Through Crisis: Polio Victims and their Families*, Bobbs-Merrill, Indianapolis, IN.

Deatrick, J.A., Stull, M.K., Dixon, D. *et al.* (1986) Measuring parent participation: Part II. *Issues in Comprehensive Pediatric Nursing*, **9**(4), 239–246.

Department of Health (1991) *Welfare of Children and Young People in Hospital*, HMSO, London.

Department of Health and Social Security (1976) *Fit For the Future (The Court Report)*, 2 vols, HMSO, London.

Diekelmann, N. (1993) Transforming RN education: New approaches to innovation, in *Transforming RN Education: Dialogue and Debate*, (eds N.L. Diekelmann and M.L. Rather), National League for Nursing, New York.

Dingwall, R. (1977) 'Atrocity stories' and professional relationships. *Sociology of Work and Occupations*, **4**(4), 371–396.

Dingwall, R. (1980) Ethics and ethnography. *Sociological Review*, **28**(4), 871–891.

Drabble, M. (1965) *The Millstone*, Weidenfeld and Nicholson, London.

Drew, N. (1986) Exclusion and confirmation: A phenomenology of patients' experiences with caregivers. *Image: Journal of Nursing Scholarship*, **18**(2), 39–43.

Dreyfus, H.L. (1983) Being in the World: A Commentary on Heidegger's 'Being and Time, Division 1'. Philosophy Department, University of California, Berkeley, CA. Mimeo.

Dreyfus, H.L. (1991) Being in the World: A Commentary on Heidegger's 'Being and Time, Division 1', MIT Press, Cambridge, MA.

Duncombe, M.A. (1951) Daily visiting in children's wards. *Nursing Times*, **47**, 587–588.

Elfert, H. and Anderson, J.M. (1987) More than just luck: Parents' views on getting good nursing care. *Canadian Nurse*, **83**(4), 14–17.

Eltzer, C.A. (1984) Parents' reactions to pediatric critical care settings: A review of the literature. *Issues in Comprehensive Pediatric Nursing*, **7**, 319–331.

Emerson, R.M. (1987) Four ways to improve the craft of fieldwork. *Journal of Contemporary Ethnography*, **16**(1), 69–89.

Fagin, C.M. and Nusbaum, J.G. (1978) Parental visiting privileges in pediatric units: A survey. *Journal of Nursing Administration*, **8**, 24–27.

Festervand, T.A. (1985) An introduction and application of focus group research to the health care industry. *Health Marketing Quarterly*, **2**(2–3), 199–209.

Field, P.A. (1981) A phenomenological look at giving an injection. *Journal of Advanced Nursing*, **6**(4), 291–296.

Field, P.A. and Morse, J.M. (1985) *Nursing Research: The Application of Qualitative Approaches*, Croom Helm, London.

Fielding, N.G. and Fielding, J.L. (1986) *Linking Data: The Articulation of Qualitative and Quantitative Methods in Social Science*, Sage Publications, London.

Fletcher, B. (1981) Psychosocial upset in post-hospitalised children: A review of the literature. *Maternal and Child Nursing Journal*, **10**, 185–195.

Foucault, M. (1973) *The Birth of the Clinic*, Tavistock Press, London.

Foucault, M. (1977) *Discipline and Punish: The Birth of the Prison*, Penguin, Harmondsworth.

Foucault, M. (1980) *Power/Knowledge: Selected Interviews and Other Writings 1972–1977*, (ed. C. Gordon), Harvester Press, Brighton.

Frank, A. (1991) *At The Will of the Body: Reflections on Illness*, Houghton Mifflin, Boston, MA.

Frank, R. (1952) Parents and the pediatric nurse. *American Journal of Nursing*, **52**(1), 76–77.

Fraser, N. (1989) *Unruly Practices: Power, Discourse and Gender in Contemporary Social Theory*, Polity Press, Cambridge.

Gadamer, H-G. (1975) *Truth and Method*, Sheed & Ward, London.

Gadamer, H-G. (1984) The hermeneutics of suspicion, in *Hermeneutics: Questions and Prospects*, (eds G. Shapiro and A. Sica), University of Massachusetts Press, Amherst, MA.

Gadow, S. (1980) Existential advocacy: Philosophical foundations of nursing, in *Nursing: Images and Ideals – Opening Dialogues with the Humanities*, (eds S.F. Spicker and S. Gadow), Springer, New York.

Gadow, S. (1985) Nurse and patient: The caring relationship, in *Caring, Curing, Coping: Nurse, Physician, Patient Relationships*, (eds A.H. Bishop and J.R. Scudder Jr), University of Alabama Press, AL.

Gadow, S. (1990) The advocacy covenant: Care as clinical subjectivity, in *Knowledge About Care and Caring: State of the Art and Future Developments*, (eds J.S. Stevenson and T. Tripp-Reimer), American Academy of Nursing, Kansas City, MO.

Gill, K.M. (1987a) Parent participation with a family health focus: Nurses' attitudes. *Pediatric Nursing*, **13**(2), 94–96.

Gill, K.M. (1987b) Nurses' attitudes toward parent participation: Personal and professional characteristics. *Children's Health Care*, **15**(3), 149–151.

Giorgi, A. (1970) *Psychology as a Human Science: A Phenomenologically Based Approach*, Harper and Row, New York.

Giorgi, A. (1975) Convergence and divergence of qualitative and quantitative methods in psychology, in *Duquesne Studies in Phenomenological Psychology, vol. II*, (eds A. Giorgi, C. Fisher and E. Murray), Duquesne University Press, Pittsburgh, PA.

Glaser, B.G. and Strauss, A.L. (1967) *The Discovery of Grounded Theory*, Aldine, Chicago, IL.

Glasper, E.A. and Tucker, A. (1993) *Advances in Child Health Nursing*, Scutari Press, London.

Goffman, E. (1959) *The Presentation of Self in Everyday Life*, Doubleday, New York.

Goodell, S.A. (1979) Perceptions of nurses toward parent participation on pediatric oncology units. *Cancer Nursing*, **2**, 38–46.

Green, M. and Green, J.G. (1977) The parent care pavilion. *Child Today*, **6**, 5–8.

Green-Hernandez, C. (1991) Professional nurse caring: A conceptual model for nursing, in *Caring and Nursing: Explorations in Feminist Perspectives*, (eds R.M. Neil and R. Watts), National League for Nursing, New York.

Guba, E.G. (1981) Criteria for assessing the trustworthiness of naturalistic inquiries. *Educational Communication and Technology Journal*, **29**(2), 75–91.

Gubrium, J.F. and Buckholdt, D.R. (1982a) Fictive family: Everyday usage, analytic and service considerations. *American Anthropologist*, **84**, 878–885.

Gubrium, J.F. and Buckholdt, D.R. (1982b) *Describing Care: Image and Practice in Rehabilitation*, Oelgeshlager, Gunn & Hain, Boston, MA.

Gubrium, J.F. and Lynott, R.J. (1985) Family rhetoric as social order. *Journal of Family Issues*, **6**(1), 129–152.

Gubrium, J.F. and Silverman, D. (1989) *The Politics of Field Research: Sociology Beyond Enlightenment*, Sage Publications, London.

Hall, D.J. (1977) *Social Relations and Innovation: Changing the State of Play in Hospitals*, Routledge & Kegan Paul, London.

Hall, D.J. (1978) Bedside blues: The impact of social research on the hospital treatment of sick children. *Journal of Advanced Nursing*, **3**(1), 25–37.

Hall, D.J. (1979) On calling for order: Aspects of the organisation of patient care, in *Beyond Separation: Further Studies of Children in Hospital*, (eds D.J. Hall and M. Stacey), Routledge & Kegan Paul, London.

Hall, D.J. (1987) Social and psychological care before and during hospitalisation. *Social Science and Medicine*, **25**(6), 721–732.

Hammersley, M. and Atkinson, P. (1983) *Ethnography: Principles in Practice*, Tavistock Press, London.

Hardgrove, C. (1980) Helping parents on the paediatric ward: A report on a survey of hospitals with 'living-in' programs. *Pediatrician*, **9**, 220–223.

Hardyment, C. (1983) *Dream Babies: Child Care from Locke to Spock*, Jonathan Cape, London.

Hartrich, P. (1956) Parents and nurses work together. *Nursing Outlook*, **4**(3), 146–148.

Hawker, R. (1984) Rules to control visitors 1746–1900. *Nursing Times (Occasional Paper)* **80**(9), 49–51.

Hawker, R. (1985) Gatekeeping: A traditional and contemporary function of the nurse, in *Political Issues in Nursing: Past, Present and Future*, (ed. R. White), John Wiley & Sons, Chichester.

Hawthorne, P.J. (1974) *Nurse – I Want My Mummy!* Royal College of Nursing, London.

Hayes, V.E. and Knox, J.E. (1984) The experience of stress in parents of children hospitalised with long term disabilities. *Journal of Advanced Nursing*, **9**(4), 333–341.

Heidegger, M. (1962) *Being and Time*, (trans. J. MacQuarrie and E. Robinson), Basil Blackwell, Oxford.

Heidegger, M. (1966) *Discourse on Thinking*, (trans. J.M. Anderson and E.H. Freund), Harper Torchbooks, New York.

Heimann-Ratain, G, Hanson, M. and Peregoy, S. (1985) The role of focus group interviews in designing a smoking prevention programme. *Journal of School Health*, **55**(1), 13–16.

Heller, A. (1984) *Everyday Life*, Routledge & Kegan Paul, London.

Hill, C. (1978) The mother on the pediatric ward: Insider or outlawed? *Pediatric Nursing*, **4**(5), 26–29.

Hilton, T. (1982) A shared experience. *World Medicine*, **18**(2), 26.

Hochschild, A.R. (1983) *The Managed Heart: The Commercialization of Human Feeling*, University of California Press, Berkeley, CA.

Hohle, B. (1957) We admit the parents too. *American Journal of Nursing*, **57**(7), 865–867.

Hunt, M. (1991) Being friendly and informal: Reflected in nurses', terminally ill patients', and relatives' conversations at home. *Journal of Advanced Nursing*, **16**(8), 929–938.

Husserl, E. (1962) *Ideas: General Introduction to Phenomenology*, Collier, New York.

Husserl, E. (1982) *Ideas Pertaining to a Pure Phenomenology and to a Phenomenological Philosophy*, Martinus Nijhoff, The Hague.

Hutchinson, S. (1986) Grounded theory: The method, in *Nursing Research: A Qualitative Perspective*, (eds P.L. Munhall and C.J. Oiler), Appleton-Century-Crofts, Norwalk, CT.

Jackson, P., Bradham, R. and Burwell, H. (1978) Child care in the hospital – a parent/staff partnership. *American Journal of Maternal Child Nursing*, **3**, 104–107.

Jacobs, R. (1979) The meaning of hospital: The denial of emotions, in *Beyond Separation: Further Studies of Children in Hospital*, (eds D.J. Hall and M. Stacey), Routledge & Kegan Paul, London.

Jick, T.D. (1979) Mixing qualitative and quantitative methods: Triangulation in action. *Administrative Science Quarterly*, **24**, 602–611.

Johnson, J.M. (1975) *Doing Field Research*, Free Press, New York.

Jolly, J. (1981) *Communicating With Children in Hospital*, H.M.& M, London.

Kasch, C. (1986) Toward a theory of nursing action. *Nursing Research*, **35**(4), 226–230.

Keane, S., Garralda, M.E. and Keen, J.H. (1986) Resident parents during paediatric admissions. *International Journal of Nursing Studies*, **23**(3), 247–253.

Kearney, R. (1986) *Modern Movements in European Philosophy*, University of Manchester Press, Manchester.

Kelly, M. and May, D. (1982) Good and bad patients: A review of the literature and a theoretical critique. *Journal of Advanced Nursing*, **7**, 147–156.

Khan, D.L. and Steeves, R.H. (1988) Caring and practice: Construction of the nurse's world. *Scholarly Inquiry for Nursing Practice*, **2**(3), 201–215.

Khoo, H. (1972) Rapport between parents and nurses in a children's ward. *Nursing Journal of Singapore*, **12**(1), 21–23.

Kierkegaard, S. (1956) *Purity of Heart is to Will One Thing*, Harper & Row, New York.

Knafl, K.A., Cavallari, K.A. and Dixon, D.M. (1988) *Pediatric Hospitalization: Family and Nurse Perspectives*, Scott, Foresman & Co., Glenview, IL.

Knafl, K.A. and Dixon, D.M. (1984) The participation of fathers in their child's hospitalisation. *Issues in Comprehensive Pediatric Nursing*, **7**(4–5), 269–281.

Knowlden, V. (1991) Nurse caring as constructed knowledge, in *Caring and Nursing: Explorations in Feminist Perspectives*, (eds R.M. Neil and R. Watts), National League for Nursing, New York.

Knox, J.E. and Hayes, V.E. (1983) Hospitalisation of a chronically ill child: A stressful time for parents. *Issues in Comprehensive Pediatric Nursing*, **6**, 217–226.

Kvale, S. (1983) The qualitative research interview: A phenomenological and a hermeneutical mode of understanding. *Journal of Phenomenological Psychology*, **14**(2), 171–196.

La Rossa, R. (1986) *Becoming a Parent*, Sage Publications, London.

Leininger, M. (1978) *Transcultural Nursing: Concepts, Theories and Practices*, John Wiley & Sons, New York.

Leininger, M. and Watson, J. (1990) *The Caring Imperative in Education*, National League for Nursing, New York.

Leonard, V.W. (1989) A Heideggerian phenomenologic perspective on the concept of the person. *Advances in Nursing Science*, **11**(4), 40–55.

Leonard, V.W. (1991) The transition to parenthood of first time mothers with career commitments: An interpretive study. Paper presented at the Qualitative Health Research Conference, February 1991, Edmonton, Alberta.

Lovell-Davis, J. (1986) When children cry alone. *Nursing Times*, **30 April**, 16–17

MacCarthy, D. and MacKeith, R. (1965) A Parent's Voice. *Lancet*, **ii**, 1289–1291.

MacDonald, E.M. (1969) Parents' preparation in care of the hospitalised child. *Canadian Nurse*, **65**, 37–39.

McIntosh, J.B. (1979) The nurse–patient relationship. *Nursing Mirror*, **148**(4), 11–20 (supplement).

MacIntyre, A. (1981) *After Virtue*, University of Notre Dame Press, Notre Dame, Quebec.

MacIntyre, S. (1979) Some issues in the study of pregnancy careers. *Sociological Review*, **27**(4), 755–771.

MacLeod, M.L.P. (1990) Experience in everyday nursing practice: A study of 'experienced' ward sisters. University of Edinburgh. PhD thesis.

McMahon, M. (1991) Nursing histories: Reviving life in abandoned selves. *Feminist Review*, **37**, 23–37.

MacQuarrie, J. (1972) *Existentialism*, Penguin, Harmondsworth.

Mahaffy, P.R. (1964) Nurse–parent relationships in living-in situations. *Nursing Forum*, **3**, 52–68.

Malinowski, B. (1922) *Argonauts of the Western Pacific*, Routledge & Kegan Paul, London.

Martin, M. (1986) Confidence not courage. *Intensive Care Nursing*, **2**(1), 20–22.

Meadow, S.R. (1969) The captive mother. *Archives of Diseases in Childhood*, **44**(3), 362–367.

Meadow, S.R. (1974) Children, mothers and hospital. *New Society*, **27**(592), 318–320.

Meleis, A.I. (1991) *Theoretical Nursing: Development and Progress*, 2nd edn, J.B. Lippincott, Philadelphia, PA.

Melia, K.M. (1981) Student nurses' accounts of their work and training: A qualitative analysis. University of Edinburgh. PhD thesis.

Melia, K.M. (1987) *Learning and Working: The Occupational Socialisation of Nurses*, Tavistock Press, London.

Meltzer, B.N., Petras, J.W. and Reynolds, L.T. (1975) *Symbolic Interactionism: Genesis, Varieties and Criticism*, Routledge & Kegan Paul, London.

Mennerick, L.A. (1974) Client typologies: A method of coping with conflict in the service worker–client relationship. *Sociology of Work and Occupations*, **1**(4), 396–418.

Menzies, I.E.P. (1967) *The Functioning of Social Systems as a Defense Against Anxiety*, Tavistock Press, London.

Merrow, D.L. and Johnson, B.S. (1968) Perceptions of the mother's role with her hospitalised child. *Nursing Research*, **17**(2), 155–156.

Miles, I. (1986a) The emergence of sick children's nursing. Part 1: Sick children's nursing before the turn of the century. *Nurse Education Today*, **6**(2), 82–87.

Miles, I. (1986b) The emergence of sick children's nursing. Part 2: Efforts and achievements in the 20th century. *Nurse Education Today*, **6**(3), 133–138.

Ministry of Health (Central Health Services Council) (1959) *The Welfare of Children in Hospital. Report of the Committee (The Platt Report)*, HMSO, London.

Mishel, M.H. (1983) Parents' perceptions of uncertainty concerning their hospitalised child. *Nursing Research*, **32**(6), 324–330.

Misiak, H. and Sexton, V.S. (1973) *Phenomenological, Existential and Humanistic Psychologies: A Historical Survey*, Grune & Stratton, New York.

Mitchell, E.S. (1986) Multiple triangulation: A methodology for nursing science. *Advances in Nursing Science*, **8**(3), 18–26.

Monahan, G.H. and Schkade, J.K. (1985) Comparing care by parent and traditional nursing units. *Pediatric Nursing*, **11**(6), 463–468,

Moran, P. (1963) Parents in pediatrics. *Nursing Forum*, **2**(3), 24–37.

Morgan, G. (1983) *Beyond Method: Strategies for Social Research*, Sage Publications, London.

Morgan, M.L. and Lloyd, B.J. (1955) Parents invited. *Nursing Outlook*, **3**(5), 256–257.

Morgan, D.L. and Spanish, M.T. (1984) Focus groups: A new tool for qualitative research. *Qualitative Sociology*, **7**(3), 253–270.

Morse, J.M. (1991) Negotiating commitment and involvement in the nurse–patient relationship. *Journal of Advanced Nursing*, **16**, 455–468.

Morse, J.M., Solberg, S.M., Neander, W.L. *et al.* (1990) Concepts of caring and caring as a concept. *Advances in Nursing Science*, **13**(1), 1–14.

Munhall, P.L. and Oiler, C.J. (eds) (1986) Nursing Research: A Qualitative Perspective, Appleton-Century-Crofts, Norwalk, CT.

National League for Nursing (1989) *Curriculum Revolution: Reconceptualising Nursing Education*, National League for Nursing, New York.

National League for Nursing (1990) *Curriculum Revolution: Redefining the Student-Teacher Relationship*, National League for Nursing, New York.

National League for Nursing (1991) *Curriculum Revolution: Community Building and Activism*, National League for Nursing. New York.

Nettleton, S. (1991) Wisdom, diligence and teeth: Discursive practices and the creation of mothers. *Sociology of Health and Illness*, **13**(1), 98–111.

Nolan, H. (1981) Hospitalisation of infants and pre-schoolers: Observations and reflections by a live-in mother. *The Lamp*, **38**(8), 29–35.

Nursing Times Editorial (1953) Editorial: The child as a person in the hospital. *Nursing Times*, **49**, 1153–1154.

Oakley, A. (1974a) *The Sociology of Housework*, Martin Robertson, Oxford.

Oakley, A. (1974b) *Housewife*, Penguin, Harmondsworth.

Orton, H. (1981) *Ward Learning Climate*, Royal College of Nursing, London.

Park, C. (1991) The involvement of parents in the care of their hospitalised child. Paper presented at the Qualitative Health Research Conference, February 1991, Edmonton, Alberta.

Parse, R.R. (1981) *Man-Living-Health: A Theory of Nursing* , John Wiley & Sons, New York.

Paterson, J.G. and Zderad, L.T. (1976) *Humanistic Nursing*, National League for Nursing, New York..

Payne, G., Dingwall, R., Payne, J. and Carter, M. (1981) *Sociology and Social Research*, Routledge & Kegan Paul, London.

Pembrey, S. (1980) *The Ward Sister – Key to Nursing*, Royal College of Nursing, London.

Pickerill, C.M. and Pickerill, H.P. (1946) Keeping mother and baby together. *British Medical Journal*, **2**, 337.

Pickerill, C.M. and Pickerill, H.P. (1954) Elimination of hospital cross-infection in children: Nursing by the mother. *Lancet*, **i**, 425–429.

Pill, R. (1970) The sociological aspects of the case-study sample, in *Hospitals, Children and Their Families*, (ed. M. Stacey), Routledge & Kegan Paul, London.

Pirsig, R. (1974) *Zen and the Art of Motorcycle Maintenance*, The Bodley Head, London.

Poslusny, S.M. (1991) Friendship as a paradigm for nursing science: Using scientific subjectivity and ethical interaction to promote understanding and social change, in *Caring and Nursing: Explorations in Feminist Perspectives*, (eds R.M. Neil and R. Watts), National League for Nursing, New York.

Rabinow, P. and Sullivan, W.M. (1979) *Interpretive Social Science: A Reader*, University of California Press, Berkeley, CA.

Reeder, F. (1987) The phenomenological movement. *Image: Journal of Nursing Scholarship*, **19**3), 150–152.

Reimen, D.J. (1982) The essential structure of a caring interaction: Doing phenomenology, in *Nursing Research: A Qualitative Perspective*, (eds P.L. Munhall and C.J. Oiler), Appleton-Century-Crofts, Norwalk, CT.

Richardson, D. (1991) *Women*, Motherhood and Childrearing, Macmillan, London.

Roach, S.R. (1987) *The Human Act of Caring: A Blueprint for the Health Professions*, Canadian Hospital Association, Ottawa.

Robbins, L.S. and Wolf, F.M. (1988) Confrontation and politeness strategies in physician–patient interactions. *Social Science and Medicine*, **27**(3), 217–221.

Robertson, J. (1962) *Hospitals and Children: A Review of Letters From Parents to 'The Observer' and the BBC*, Victor Gollancz, London.

Robertson, J. (1970) *Young Children in Hospital*, 2nd edn, Tavistock Press, London.

Robertson, J. and Robertson, J. (1989) *Separation and the Very Young*, Free Association Books, London.

Robinson, C.A. (1985) Parents of hospitalised chronically ill children: Competency in question. *Nursing Papers*, **17**(2), 59–67.

Robinson, C.A. (1987) Roadblocks to family centred care when a chronically ill child is hospitalised. *Maternal Child Nursing Journal*, **16**(3), 181–193.

Robinson, C.A. and Thorne, S. (1984) Strengthening family 'interference'. *Journal of Advanced Nursing*, **9**(6), 597–602.

Rodgers, R. (1980) *From Crowther to Warnock: How 14 Reports Tried to Change Children's Lives*, Heinemann Educational Books, London.

Rubin, J. (1984) Too Much of Nothing: Modern Culture, the Self and Salvation in Kierkegaard's Thought. University of California at San Francisco. PhD thesis.

Ruddick, S. (1989) *Maternal Thinking: Toward a Politics of Peace*, Beacon Press, Boston, MA.

Sainsbury, C.P.Q., Gray, O.P., Cleary, J. *et al.* (1986) Care by parents of their children in hospital. *Archives of Disease in Childhood*, **61**(6), 612–615.

Sandelowski, M. (1986) The problem of rigour in qualitative research. *Advances in Nursing Science*, **8**(3), 27–37.

Schatzman, L. and Strauss, A.L. (1973) *Field Research: Strategies for a Natural Sociology*, Prentice-Hall, Englewood Cliffs, NJ.

Schleiermacher, F. (1977) *Hermeneutics: The Handwritten Manuscripts*, (ed. H. Kimmerle), Scholars' Press, Atlanta, GA.

Scott, D.W., Oberst, M.T. and Dropkin, M.J. (1980) A stress–coping model. *Advances in Nursing Science*, **3**, 9–23.

Seamon, D. (1984) Phenomenologies of environment and place. Phenomenology and Pedagogy, **2**(2), 130–135.

Seidl, F. and Pilliterri, A. (1967) Development of an attitude scale on parent participation. *Nursing Research*, **16**, 71–73.

Seidl, F.W. (1969) Pediatric nursing personnel and parent participation: A study in attitudes. *Nursing Research*, **18**(1), 40–44.

Selye, H. (1976) *Stress in Health and Disease*, Butterworth, London.

Shelton, T., Jeppson, E. and Johnson, B. (1987) *Family Centred Care for Children With Special Health Care Needs*, Association for the Care of Children's Health, Washington, DC.

Silverman, D. (1985) *Qualitative Methodology and Sociology*, Gower, Aldershot.

Silverman, D. (1987) *Communication and Medical Practice: Social Relations in the Clinic*, Sage Publications, London.

Silverman, D. (1989) Telling convincing stories: A plea for cautious positivism in case studies, in *The Qualitative–Quantitative Distinction in the Social Sciences*, (eds B. Glassner and J.D. Moreno), Kluwer Academic Publishers, Dordrecht.

Skidmore, D. (1986) The Sociology of Friendship: Historical, literary and Empirical Perspectives. University of Keele. PhD thesis.

Smart, B. (1985) *Michel Foucault*, Tavistock Press, London.

Smith, R. (1980) Skepticism and qualitative research. *Education and Urban Society*, **12**(3), 383–389.

Smith, S.J. (1989) Operating on a child's heart: A pedagogical view of hospitalisation. *Phenomenology and Pedagogy*, **7**, 145–162.

Smith, S.M. (1987) Primary nursing in the NICU: A parent's perspective. *Neonatal Network*, **5**(4), 25–27.

Smith, J.K. and Heshusius, L. (1986) Closing down the conversation: the end of the quantitative–qualitative debate among educational researchers. *Educational Researcher*, **15**, 4–12.

Sosnowitz, B.G. (1984) Managing parents on neonatal ICUs. *Social Problems*, **31**(4), 390–402.

Spence, J.C. (1946) *The Purpose of the Family: A Guide to the Care of Children*, National Children's Homes, London.

Spiegelberg, H. (1982) *The Phenomenological Movement*, 3rd edn, Martinus Nijhoff, The Hague.

Spradley, J.P. (1979) *The Ethnographic Interview*, Holt, Rinehart & Winston, New York.

Spradley, J.P. (1980) *Participant Observation*, Rinehart and Winston, New York.

Stacey, M. (1979) The practical implications of our conclusions, in *Beyond Separation: Further Studies of Children in Hospital*, (eds D.J. Hall and M. Stacey), Routledge & Kegan Paul, London.

Stacey, M., Batstone, E., Bell, C. and Murcott, A. (1975) Power, Persistence and Change: A Second Study of Banbury, Routledge & Kegan Paul, London.

Stacey, M., Dearden, R., Pill, R. and Robinson, D. (1970) Hospitals, Children and Their Families: The Report of a Pilot Study, Routledge & Kegan Paul. London.

Stern, P.N., Allen, L.M. and Moxley, P.A. (1984) Qualitative research: The nurse as a grounded theorist. *Health Care for Women International*, **5**(5–6), 371–385.

Strauss, A.L. (1987) *Qualitative Analysis for Social Scientists*, Cambridge University Press, Cambridge.

Strong, P.M. (1979a) *The Ceremonial Order of the Clinic: Parents, Doctors and Medical Bureaucracies*, Routledge & Kegan Paul, London.

Strong, P.M. (1979b) Sociological imperialism and the profession of medicine. *Social Science and Medicine*, **13A**, 199–215.

Stull, M.K. and Deatrick, J.A. (1986) Measuring parental participation: Part I. *Issues in Comprehensive Pediatric Nursing*, **9**(3), 157–165.

Swanson, J.M. (1986) The formal qualitative interview for grounded theory, in *From*

Practice to Grounded Theory, (eds W.C. Chenitz and J.M. Swanson), Addison-Wesley, Menlo Park, CA.

Swanson-Kauffman, K.M. (1986) A combined qualitative methodology for nursing research. *Advances in Nursing Science*, **8**(3), 58–69.

Swanwick, M. (1983) Platt in perspective. *Nursing Times (Occasional Paper)*, **79**(2), 5–8.

Taylor, C. (1985a) *Human Agency and Language: Philosophical Papers 1*, Cambridge University Press, Cambridge.

Taylor, C. (1985b) Theories of meaning, in *Human Agency and Language: Philosophical Papers 1*, (ed. C. Taylor), Cambridge University Press, Cambridge.

Taylor, C. (1989) *Sources of the Self: The Making of the Modern Identity*, Cambridge University Press, Cambridge.

Thorne, S.E. and Robinson, C.A. (1988a) Reciprocal trust in health care relationships. *Journal of Advanced Nursing*, **13**(6), 782–789.

Thorne, S.E. and Robinson, C.A. (1988b) Health care relationships: The chronic illness perspective. *Research in Nursing and Health*, **11**(5), 293–300.

Thornes, R. (1983a) Parental access and family facilities in children's wards in England. *British Medical Journal* , **287**, 190–192.

Thornes, R. (1983b) Parental access and overnight accommodation in childrens' wards in England: The regional picture. National Association for the Welfare of Children in Hospital (NAWCH), London. Mimeo.

Thornes, R. (1987) *Parents Staying Overnight With Their Children in Hospital*, National Association for the Welfare of Children in Hospital (NAWCH), London.

Tofias, L. (1989) Expert practice: Trading examples over pizza. *American Journal of Nursing*, **89**(9), 1193–1194.

Travelbee, J. (1971) *Interpersonal Aspects of Nursing*, 2nd edn, F.A. Davis, Philadelphia, PA.

Turner, J. (1984) A parent's perspective. *Nursing Mirror*, **159**(18), 23–25.

Van Manen, M. (1990) *Researching Lived Experience: Human Science for an Action Sensitive Pedagogy*, Althouse Press, Ontario.

Warshay, L.H. and Warshay, D.W. (1987) Symbolic interactionism: Humanists versus positivists. *International Social Science Review*, **62**(2), 51–66.

Waterhouse, R. (1981) *A Heidegger Critique: A Critical Examination of the Existential Philosophy of Martin Heidegger*, Harvester Press, Brighton.

Watson, J. (1979) *Nursing: The Philosophy and Science of Caring*, Little, Brown & Co., Boston, MA.

Watson, J. (1985) *Nursing: Human Science and Human Care*, a Theory of Nursing, Appleton-Century-Crofts, Norwalk, CT.

Watson, J. (1988a) *Nursing: Human Science and Human Care*, revised reprint, National League For Nursing, New York.

Watson, J. (1988b) Response to 'Caring and practice: Construction of the nurse's world'. *Scholarly Inquiry for Nursing Practice*, **2**(3), 217–221.

Webb, B. (1977) Trauma and tedium, in *Medical Encounters: The Experience of Illness and Treatment*, (eds A. Davis and G. Horobin), Croom Helm, London.

Webb, N., Hull, D. and Madeley, R. (1985) Care by parents in hospital. *British Medical Journal*, **291**(6489), 176–177.

Wolfe, L. (1985) Parental access and family facilities in wards admitting children in Scotland. National Association for the Welfare of Children in Hospital (NAWCH), London. Mimeo.

Wollcott, H.F. (1990) *Writing up Qualitative Research*, Sage Publications, London.

Zerubavel, E. (1979) *Patterns of Time in Hospital Life*, University of Chicago Press, Chicago, IL.

Index

Action for Sick Children, *see* NAWCH
Adamson, E.F. 35
Admission to hospital 17, 23, 24, 25, 140
Agan, R.D. 107
Algren, C.L. 8
Allan, G. 169
Allen, D.G. 40, 165, 190
Anderson, J.M. 1
Anonymous 15
Anstice, E. 10
Arango, P. 15
Archbold, P. 202
Armitage, S. 45, 50
Armstrong, G. xvii, 2
    see also Miles, I.
Athens, L.H. 187
Atkinson, P. 204, 205

Baruch, G. 63, 69, 116
Beardslee, W.R. 74
Beck, L. 7, 200
Becker, H. 201
Beckett, J. 14, 15
Being-in-the-world 191, 192
Bell, C. 12
Bellah, R.N. 16
Benner, P. 9, 11, 16, 23, 33, 74, 81, 97,
    107, 120, 126, 129, 137, 139, 146,
    163, 165, 166, 168, 172, 174, 175,
    176, 177, 179, 181, 182, 183, 186,
    189, 190
    see also 'Deficit mode' thinking;
    Technocure model
Bentham, J. 173
Bergum,V. 133, 167
Berman, D.C. 10
Betz, C.L. 89
Beuf, A.H. 11, 146, 172

Bevis, E.O. 184
Bishop, A.H. 162, 163, 179, 184
Bleicher, J. 16, 183, 187
Bloor, M.J. 205, 206
Blumer, H. 191, 192, 193, 197
Bogdan, R. 74
Bollnow, O.F. 168
Bordo, S. 165
Borman, K.M. 205
Boulton, M.G. 166
Bowers, B.J. 192
Bowlby, J. 3
Brain, D.J. 10
Brink, P.J. 187
Brossat, S. 81
Brown, J. 7, 102, 196
Brunvand, J.H. 63
Buber, M. 162, 163
Buckholdt, D.R. 46, 49, 51, 53, 69, 71
Burgess, R.G. 195

Calder, B. 199
Callery, P. 172
Care By Parent Unit 7
Caring xvii, 2, 15, 48, 61, 62, 63, 108,
    117, 120, 125, 127, 129, 135, 136,
    137, 163, 171, 175, 176, 177, 180,
    183, 184
Caring practices 175, 177, 181
    distinguished from behaviours 124
Carpenter, S. 56
Chopoorian, T. 168
Cleary, J. 1, 102
Cohen, M.Z. 190
Connectedness 38, 115, 127, 133, 134,
    135, 144, 153, 154, 162, 180
    defined 127
Consumers Association 1, 5

Coucouvanis, J.A. 46
Craik, J. 174
Crow, G. 169

DHSS, *see* Department of Health and
    Social Security
Darbyshire, P. 185
Davis, B. 26, 139
De Maso, D.R. 74
Deatrick, J.A. 8
'Deficit mode' thinking 11
Demarcation of care 109, 110, 113
Department of Health xvii, 89
Department of Health and Social Security
    5
Diekelmann, N. 182
Dilthey, W. 187, 192
Dingwall, R. 63, 201, 203
Discipline 18, 35, 36, 37, 114, 169, 174
Dixon, D. 8, 47, 195
Drabble, M. 4
Drew, N. 133, 191
Dreyfus, H.L. 13, 16, 81, 168, 193
Duncombe, M. 3

Elfert, H. 1
Eliot, T.S. 182
Eltzer, C.A. 57
Emerson, R.M. 193

Fagin, C.M. 1
Family and friends 52, 146, 147, 149,
    150
Family centred care xiii, xiv, xviii, 46, 50,
    51, 52, 103, 110, 183, 187
Fathers 8, 27, 47, 48, 97, 147, 148, 149,
    158, 195
Festervand, T.A. 200
Field, P.A. 191, 194, 195
Fielding, N.G. and J.L. 189
Fletcher, B. 1
Foucault, M. 37, 172, 173, 174, 175, 201
    capillary power 174
    disciplinary gaze 37
    the 'gaze' 173, 174, 175
    'medical gaze' 37
Frank, A. 5, 81
Fraser, N. 173, 175
Fusion of horizons 168, 184

Gadamer, H-G. 119, 168, 184, 185, 206
Gadow, S. 129, 136, 177
Gill, K.M. 9

Giorgi, A. 187, 190
Glaser, B.G. 14, 204, 207
Glasper, E.A. 185
Goffman, E. 11, 114
Goodell, S.A. 9
Government Reports
    Court Report 5
    Platt Report xiii, 3, 5, 6, 9, 15
    *Welfare of Children and Young People
    in Hospital* xvii
Green, M. and J.G. 7
Green-Hernandez, C. 179
Grounded theory 12, 14, 189, 190, 191,
    204, 206
Guba, E.G. 187, 193
Gubrium, J.F. 46, 47, 48, 49, 50, 51, 53,
    69, 71, 174

Hall, D.J. 1, 6, 10, 12, 89
Hammersley, M. 204, 205
Hardgrove, C. 1
Hardyment, C. 2
Hartrich, P. 5
Hawker, R. 194
Hawthorne, P.J. 3, 7, 9, 10, 109
Hayes, V.E. 12, 13, 117
Health Care Relationships Project 13, 14
Heidegger, M. 13, 17, 25, 31, 33, 35, 120,
    165, 166, 168, 176, 177, 182, 184,
    190, 192, 197, 207
    ready-to-hand 33, 35, 53
    'thrownness' 31, 53
    unready-to-hand 33
Heimann-Ratain, G. 200
Heller, A. 169
Hermeneutic circle 184, 204
Heshusius, L. 194
Hill, C. 8
Hilton, T. 14, 15
Hochschild, A.R. 44, 45
Hohle, B. 5
Home 24, 25, 58, 92, 93, 103, 109, 113,
    114, 146, 149, 150, 168, 169, 170
Hope 128, 147, 159
Hull, D. 35
Hunt, M. 179
Husserl, E. 165, 192, 197
Hutchinson, S. 191

I – It 162
I – Thou 162, 163
    see also Buber, M.
Interactional comportment 161

Jackson, P. 7
Jacobs, R. 8
Jick, T.D. 189
Johnson, B.S. 7
Johnson, J.M. 204
Jolly, J. 89

Kasch, C. 189
Keane, S. 9
Kearney, R. 192
Keeping vigil 60, 97, 98, 99, 147
Kelly, M. 55, 73, 74
Khan, D.L. 177, 178
Khoo, H. 15
Kierkegaard, S. 54, 192
King, T. 2
Knafl, K.A. 8, 47, 146, 166, 195
Knowlden, V. 179
Knowledge value differential 68, 95
Knox, J.E. 12, 13, 117
Kubler-Ross, E. 14
Kvale, S. 197

La Rossa, R. 166
Leininger, M. 184, 189
Length of stay 137, 141, 142, 144, 162,
    170, 178
Leonard, V.W. 133
Lived experience 9, 16, 165, 167, 187,
    188, 190, 191
  defined 186
Lived space 168
Lived world 192
Lloyd, B.J. 5
Lovell-Davis, J. 43
Lynott, R.J. 46, 47, 48

MacCarthy, D. 3, 4
MacDonald, E.M. 7
McIntosh, J.B. 169
MacIntyre, A. 124
MacIntyre, S. 188
MacKeith, R. 4
MacLay, I. 10
MacLeod, M.L.P. 11, 175
McMahon, M. 165
MacQuarrie, J. 168
Mahaffy, P.R. 10
Malinowski, B. 197
Managerialism 184
Martin, M. 15
Maternal deprivation 3
May, D. 55, 73, 74

Meadow, R. 6, 9, 97, 99, 166
Meals and breaks 48, 58, 59, 64, 81, 98,
    99, 102, 142, 147
Meleis, A.I. 182
Melia, K.M. 26, 102, 109, 122, 124, 191
Meltzer, B.N. 192
Mennerick, L.A. 77
Menzies, I.E.P. 124
Merleau-Ponty, M. 192
Merrow, D.L. 7
Miles, I. xvii, 2
Ministry of Health 1, 5
Mishel, M.H. 31
Misiak, H. 191, 192
Mitchell, E.S. 189
Monaghan, G.H. 7
Moran, P. 10
Morgan, G. 188, 199
Morgan, M.L. 5
Morris, I. 3
Morse, J.M. 127, 135, 139, 176, 180, 181,
    194, 195
Mothers' Unit 24, 48, 54, 63, 64, 98, 156,
    160
Munhall, P.L. 191

NAWCH (National Association for the
    Welfare of Children in Hospital) 6
National League for Nursing 184
Nettleton, S. 172
Newby, H. 12
Nightingale, F. 5
Nolan, H. 14
Nurse–parent relationships xiv, 1, 9, 11,
    13, 16, 47, 72, 75, 81, 110, 120, 125,
    133, 136, 139, 162, 176
Nurses
  assessments of parents 18, 43, 44, 62,
    72, 106, 134, 139
    intuitive 107, 108
  'busyness' 19, 38, 65, 102, 122
  caring practices 80, 124, 125, 127, 128,
    129, 136, 137, 162, 164, 174, 175,
    176, 179,
    183
  expectations of parents 69
  individual v. universal concerns 103,
    138
  the personal and the
    professional 129
  professional detachment 131, 136
  professional identity 115, 117
  who were also parents 132

Nursing Times 5
Nusbaum, J.G. 1

Oakley, A. 169
Oiler, C.J. 191
Orton, H. 196

Panopticon 173, 174
Parent participation xiii, xiv, xvii,
    xviii, 6, 7, 8, 9, 46, 52, 66, 73,
    83, 92, 93, 104, 108, 172, 176,
    183
  fathers 9, 12, 47
Parenting in public xiii, 16, 17, 35,
    126, 161, 168, 169
Parents
  arguments against daily visiting 3
  asking 'stupid' questions 45
  basic mothering 42, 43, 45, 48, 67,
    83, 87, 93, 94, 96, 103, 109, 110,
    112, 143
  being 'all in the same boat' 153,
    155, 160, 164
  being on the 'wrong side' of staff
    63
  being-in-the-world 13, 17, 33, 53,
    120, 133, 167, 185
  confidence 7, 65, 67, 68, 117,
    132
  distress 19, 22, 24, 132, 156, 160
  encouraging participation 1, 181
  expert parents 84, 104, 115, 116,
    117
  feelings of guilt 14, 23, 32, 53, 55,
    57, 65, 66, 80, 82, 99, 101, 157,
    161
  idealized view 55, 56, 61, 161
  individuality 41, 164
  information seeking 26, 62, 93
  intelligence 44, 45, 73, 108
  'lazy' mother 10, 68
  moral identity 37, 54, 55, 57, 60,
    62, 64, 67
  'neurotic' mother 10, 62, 63, 75,
    171
  nurses' helpers 87, 96, 103, 118
  on 'the emotional roller-coaster' 31
  on the 'good side' of staff 89
  ontological understanding of xviii,
    12, 33, 53, 80, 133, 166, 167,
    168, 185
  other children 135, 146, 147, 148,
    149, 151

personality 41, 55, 73, 75, 139,
    140, 141, 163
  privacy 152, 170
  problem parents 10, 44, 50, 69, 72,
    143
  resistance to living-in 10
  resistance to visiting 3, 4, 5, 6
  sensible 71
  sexual relationships 70
  'troublemaker' 10
  uncertainty 14, 17, 23, 25, 26, 27,
    28, 29, 31, 32, 37, 40, 53, 61,
    68, 84, 85
Park, C. 133
Parse, R.R. 189
Paterson, J.G. 184, 188, 189
Payne, G. 11
Pembrey, S. 196
Phenomenology 9, 14, 16, 40, 70, 133,
    166, 167, 170, 181, 182, 184, 189,
    190, 191, 192, 197, 204, 206, 207
Pickerill, C.M. and H.P. 3
Pill, R. 11, 124
Pilliterri, A. 9
Pinell, P. 81
Pirsig, R. 165, 181, 182
Play 89
  as diversionary tactic 91
  as way of monitoring child's
    condition 92
  meaning of for parents 91, 92
  normalizing function 91
Poslusny, S.M. 179, 180
Poster, E.C. 89
Power 34, 37, 80, 102, 115, 172, 173,
    174, 175, 183, 201
  Foucault, M. and capillary power
    174
Presencing 86, 159

Rabinow, P. 16, 207
Reeder, F. 190
Reimen, D.J. 97, 191
Richardson, D. 55
Ritchie, J.A. 7
Roach, S.R. 120, 137, 162, 178
Robertson, J. and J. 1, 3, 4, 14, 15
Robertson, James
  Films
    *A Two-Year-Old Goes to
      Hospital* 3
    *John: Nine Days in a Residential
      Nursery* 3

Robbins, L.S. 62
Robinson, C.A. 13, 14, 63, 117, 146, 172
Rodgers, R. 5
Role theory 12, 13
Rubin, J. 167
Ruddick, S. 55, 167, 169, 171

Sainsbury, C.P.Q. 1, 7
Sandelowski, M. 187
Schatzman, L. 207
Schkade, J.K. 7
Schleiermacher, F. 204
Scott, D.W. 13
Scudder, J.R. Jr 162, 163, 179, 184
Seamon, D. 168
Seidl, F.W. 9
Selye, H. 13
Sexton, V.S. 191, 192
Shelton 50
Silverman, D. 40, 61, 63, 174, 182, 194,
    196, 204, 205, 206
Skidmore, D. 179, 180
Smart, B. 201
Smith, J.K. 194
Smith, L. 172
Smith, R. 188
Smith, S.J. 50
Smith, S.M. 15
Solomons, H.C. 46
Sosnowitz, B.G. 74
Spanish, M.T. 199
Special relationships 133, 135, 143,
    179
Spence, J.C. 3
Spiegelberg, H. 190
Spradley, J.P. 196, 198
Stacey, M. 10, 12, 13
Steeves, R.H. 177, 178
Stern, P.N. 191
Strauss, A.L. 14, 197, 204, 207
Strong, P.M. 12, 25, 45, 61, 63, 182, 205
Stull, M.K. 8
Sullivan, W.M. 16, 207

Swansea studies 10, 11
    see also Hall, D.J.; Jacobs, R.;
    Pill, R.; Stacey, M.
Swanson, J.M. 196
Swanson-Kauffman, K.M. 190
Swanwick, M. 5

Tanner, C. 107
Taylor, C. 9, 16, 81, 124, 165, 167, 206
Technocure model 146
Technological understanding 9, 15, 81,
    184
'The Captive Mother' 6
Thorne, S.E. 12, 13, 14, 146
Thornes, R. 6, 43
Tofias, L. 185
Travelbee, J. 189
Triangulation 189
Tucker, A. 185
Turner, J. 14, 15

Unofficial parent groups 152

Van Manen, M. 133, 165, 167, 168, 169,
    170, 182

Ward kitchen 29, 38, 39, 85, 114, 138,
    170, 173
Warshay, L.H. and D.W. 192
Waterhouse, R. 192
Watson, J.B. 2
Watson, J. 120, 177, 178, 184, 188, 189
Webb, B. 15, 163, 164, 172
Webb, N. 7, 96
Wollcott, H.F. 183
Wolf, F.M. 63
Wolfe, L. 6
Wood, M.J. 187
Wrubel, J. 23, 33, 74, 97, 120, 129, 163,
    166, 167, 168, 172, 177, 179, 183

Zderad, L.T. 184, 188, 189
Zerubavel, E. 34